T0356105

THE
LYMPHATIC
SYSTEM
HANDBOOK

THE LYMPHATIC SYSTEM HANDBOOK

Proven Lymphatic Drainage
Massage Techniques and
At-Home Strategies
for **Reducing Inflammation**
and **Managing Chronic Ailments**

FLAVIO GAZZOLA

ULYSSES PRESS

First published in 2022 in Ireland as *Masaje y Linfodrenaje* by De Vecchi Ediciones.

This English translation is published by Ulysses Press under license from Confidential Concepts International Limited.

Published in the US by:
ULYSSES PRESS
PO Box 3440
Berkeley, CA 94703
www.ulyssespress.com

ISBN: 978-1-64604-785-7
Library of Congress Control Number: 2024945009

Printed in the United States
10 9 8 7 6 5 4 3 2 1

Acquisitions editor: Casie Vogel
Managing editor: Claire Chun
US copy editor: Mark Woodworth
Proofreader: Sherian Brown
Front cover design: Rebecca Lown
Interior design and layout: Winnie Liu

NOTE TO READERS: This book has been written and published strictly for informational and educational purposes only. It is not intended to serve as medical advice or to be any form of medical treatment. You should always consult your physician before altering or changing any aspect of your medical treatment and/or undertaking a diet and/or exercise regimen, including the guidelines as described in this book. Do not stop or change any prescription medications without the guidance and advice of your physician. Any use of the information in this book is made on the reader's good judgment after consulting with his or her physician and is the reader's sole responsibility. This book is not intended to diagnose or treat any medical condition and is not a substitute for a physician.

CONTENTS

INTRODUCTION 1

SECTION 1: THE LYMPH AND
THE LYMPHATIC SYSTEM

Chapter 1
GENERAL 5
HISTORICAL TABLE.. 5
FORMATION OF THE LYMPHATIC SYSTEM............................ 6
LYMPHOID TISSUE CENTERS AND LYMPHOCYTES IN THE BLOOD 7
CLASSIFICATION OF LYMPH..7

Chapter 2
THE BASIC SYSTEM OR *GRUNDSYSTEM* 17
THE CELL.. 17
THE *GRUNDSYSTEM*..18
GRUNDSYSTEM PATHOLOGIES 20
THE DIAGNOSIS 21
THE PHASES OF THE DISEASE..22
THERAPY AND HEALING 23

Chapter 3
LYMPH CIRCULATION 25
MICROCIRCULATION 25
LYMPHATIC CAPILLARIES 26

FROM LYMPHATIC CAPILLARIES TO LYMPHATIC DUCTS.....................27

THE LYMPHATIC VESSELS 28

LYMPH CIRCULATION... 29

THE LYMPHATIC PATHWAY... 30

LEGS 31

THE PELVIS 33

THE ABDOMEN... 34

THE THORAX...37

THE ARMS... 43

THE HEAD.. 44

THE SHOULDERS..47

Chapter 4
THE LYMPH NODES 49

GENERAL 49

SECTION 2: HOW TO KEEP THE LYMPHATIC SYSTEM IN SHAPE

Chapter 5
LYMPHATIC DRAINAGE 67

GENERAL 67

CONTRAINDICATIONS 68

EFFECTS OF DRAINAGE.. 68

MAIN CLINICAL INDICATIONS FOR LYMPHATIC DRAINAGE 72

DRAINAGE TECHNIQUE 76

MECHANICAL AND ELECTRICAL MEANS FOR LYMPHATIC
DRAINAGE 79

Chapter 6
HOW TO PERFORM MANUAL LYMPHATIC DRAINAGE........ 81

Chapter 7
LYMPHATIC CIRCULATION AND WELL-BEING 155

THE SEVEN MAIN RULES 155

FOOD 156

THE DREAM 157

PHYSIOLOGICAL NEEDS.. 158

PHYSICAL AND MANUAL ACTIVITY, MEDITATION, SOCIAL LIFE,
AND SEXUALITY 159

Chapter 8
CELLULITE 161

GENERAL 161

CELLULITE CAUSED BY MENSTRUAL CYCLE IRREGULARITIES 163

CELLULITE DUE TO A SEDENTARY LIFESTYLE 164

MEANS OF CELLULITE PREVENTION AND REDUCTION 166

LYMPHATIC SELF-DRAINAGE... 170

Chapter 9
HOW TO AVOID LEG AND CHEST DISCOMFORT.............. 175

LYMPHOVENOUS INSUFFICIENCY IN THE LEGS................................ 175

LYMPHATIC STASIS OF THE BREAST 177

Chapter 10
BACK PAIN AND NEURO-LYMPHATIC TREATMENT 179

HOW TO DETECT THE AREAS TO BE MASSAGED............................. 179

BACK MASSAGE AS A COUPLE..180

SECTION 3: LYMPH DRAINAGE
AND NATURAL MEDICINE

Chapter 11
LYMPHATIC CIRCULATION AND ACUPUNCTURE 185

CHINESE ACUPUNCTURE.. 185

VOLL'S ELECTRO-ACUPUNCTURE (EAV) 186

MERIDIANS AND THE LYMPHATIC MERIDIAN................................. 187

Chapter 12
LYMPHATIC CIRCULATION AND HOMEOPATHY.............. 201

HISTORY AND PRINCIPLES OF HOMEOPATHY 201

SCHÜSSLER SALTS 206

Chapter 13
LYMPH AND PHYTOTHERAPY 211
GEMMOTHERAPY 211
A GEMMOTHERAPY RECIPE AGAINST CELLULITE 213
PHYTOTHERAPY 213
EXTERNAL-USE CREAMS AGAINST CELLULITE 214
VEGETABLE JUICES AND WFPS 217
SEAWEED 217

Chapter 14
LYMPH AND BACH FLOWERS 219
BACH FLOWER THERAPY 219
THE EFFECTS OF THE PSYCHE ON DISEASE AND VICE VERSA 220
LYMPHATIC STASIS AND EMOTIONS 220
BACH FLOWERS AND LYMPHATIC STASIS 222

Chapter 15
LYMPHATIC CIRCULATION REPRESENTED IN THE IRIS 227
BRIEF PRESENTATION OF IRIDOLOGY 227
IRIS STRUCTURE 228
THE REPRESENTATION OF THE LYMPHATIC SYSTEM IN THE IRIS 229
IRIDOPHOTOCHROMOTHERAPY 229

INDEX 231

ABOUT THE AUTHOR 240

INTRODUCTION

Lymph is the least-known fluid in the human body, even though it has three very important functions in the body. In fact, the lymphatic system is:

- The body's purification system;
- The seat of immune activity, i.e., the body's ability to defend itself;
- One of the systems responsible for physical beauty.

Lymph enables assimilation and elimination exchanges at the cellular level. The lymph carries the nutrients that reach the cells; it also carries the waste produced by cellular metabolism. After being loaded, it is filtered by structures called *lymph nodes*, and finally, at about shoulder height, it enters the venous blood stream.

Thus, poor circulation or stagnation of lymph leads to various cellular disorders due to insufficient discharge of waste, as would be the case in a city where public transport, grocery shops, and the street-cleaning service are on strike. If the stagnation is considerable, the tissues in question swell or the lymph nodes grow to the size of hazelnuts.

By contrast, if lymphatic stagnation occurs slowly or tends to be chronic, the symptoms are more confusing: tiredness, dullness of the complexion, even premature aging of the tissues. In particular, joints are affected by osteoarthritis, arteries harden (arteriosclerosis), venous vessels lose function, varicose veins appear in the lower limbs, hemorrhoids occur, and subcutaneous tissues present various problems such as cellulite.

If the stagnation is particularly severe and long-lasting, degenerative, allergic, and even autoimmune diseases as well as tumors may develop.

On the contrary, when lymph formation and circulation are regular, the body stays young, healthy, and beautiful.

The purpose of this book is to show how you can achieve and maintain this result, by illustrating the main elements of a discipline that has often been neglected.

After a first theoretical part, which deals with the characteristics of the immune system, the second part, being of a practical nature, describes the various techniques, and explains some simple drainage methods, including the treatment of cellulite and a massage that can be practiced individually or in pairs. Finally, the third part discusses the most common natural medicine remedies (phytotherapy, homeopathy, acupuncture, Bach flowers, iridology) to solve not only lymphatic stasis, but also the psychological and emotional problems resulting from it.

Section 1

THE LYMPH AND THE LYMPHATIC SYSTEM

Chapter 1

GENERAL

HISTORICAL TABLE

Gaspare Aselli (1581–1626), a surgeon and anatomist from Cremona, Italy, discovered the lymphatic vessels and described them in his book *De lactibus sive lateis venis*, named after what he thought was the milky aspect of the lymph.

Some decades later, in 1652, Thomas Bartholin determined one of the most important points of the lymphatic system: the outlet of the thoracic duct into the subclavian vein.

Since then, anatomists have used stained fluids and contrast methods to uncover lymphatic networks, as well as radioimmunological methods to study lymph nodes, in addition to techniques involving light and electron microscopy. All these have facilitated the understanding of the lymphatic system.

Today, lymphography, through the use of low-toxic chemicals, allows direct examination of a patient's lymphatic system. It is a risky examination and is therefore only recommended when other diagnostic methods are not sufficient to determine the exact nature of the problems in the lymphatic system—as may be the case, for example, before the removal of a tumor. Electro-acupuncture or EAV is another widely used method. It was developed in the 1950s, entails no risks, and enables the functionality of the lymphatic system to be precisely examined (see page 186).

FORMATION OF THE LYMPHATIC SYSTEM

The lymphatic system belongs to the circulatory system and, like that system, derives partly from the mesoderm (one of the three layers of the embryo, in which the cells of a forming organism are joined together) and partly from mesenchyme (the undifferentiated tissue, of indefinite function, that even in adults retains the possibility of transforming itself, depending on circumstances, into a certain type of tissue). Important features of this mesenchymal origin are found in the cells that make up the reticulum (the warp) and endothelium (the inner surface) of immunocompetent (body-defense) organs, such as lymph nodes, the lymph sinus, and the interior of lymphatic vessels.

The cells of the reticulum, in fact, in case of bacterial, viral, or other aggression, can transform into macrophages capable of destroying the pathogen (see the chapter on lymph nodes on page 49).

All lymphatic vessels are likely derived from the diverticula of the veins, called *lymphatic sacs*. When the embryo has reached 2 cm in length it has the following:

- two symmetrical pairs, originating from the jugular vein, and called *jugular sacs* for this reason;
- two caudal sacs derived from the iliac veins and called *iliac sacs*;
- a medium-sized sac, close to the posterior abdominal wall, called the *retroperitoneal sac*.

The beginning of the thoracic duct starts from the retroperitoneal sac and the iliac sacs. From the jugular sacs, on the other hand, depart the subclavian, the jugular, and the bronchomediastinal trunks.

Lymph nodes originate from small clusters of lymph cells along the lymphatic vessels.

The position of the parts of the lymphatic system that have already been mentioned is illustrated in the diagrams contained in the chapter on circulation (see page 25).

LYMPHOID TISSUE CENTERS AND LYMPHOCYTES IN THE BLOOD

Lymphatic tissue makes up approximately 1% of the total body weight and is primarily involved in immune defense. The lymphatic tissue centers in the body are:

- the spleen;
- the scam;
- the tonsils (palatine, pharyngeal, tubal, and lingual);
- the Peyer's patches (in the alimentary canal);
- the appendix (a real intestinal "tonsil");
- the bone marrow (to a lesser extent).

In the blood, lymphocytes (cells for the defense of the body, produced by the lymphatic tissues) make up at least 30% of the white blood cells, which in turn have a ratio of 1:1,000 to red blood cells. In one cubic millimeter of blood, therefore, there are approximately 4 to 5 million red blood cells and 4 to 5 thousand white blood cells.

CLASSIFICATION OF LYMPH

There are different types of lymph, depending on their composition and functions:

- interstitial lymph or histolymph: it is present in tissues and forms the interstitial fluid, which is the medium in which cells live (just as air is the medium in which we humans live);
- circulatory lymph: the lymph itself, which is further divided into peripheral lymph, intermediate lymph, and central lymph.

INTERSTITIAL LYMPH OR HISTOLYMPH

APPEARANCE AND FUNCTIONS

On an empty stomach, interstitial lymph is a clear, yellowish liquid with a certain viscosity, as it contains proteins and hematic cells (red blood cells, white blood cells, and so forth).

After eating, the lymph, particularly in the intestinal area, takes on a milky appearance due to the presence of fatty microglobules.

Histolymph plays a role in balancing the body's fluids. It is also a first filter for pollutants and infectious agents, which makes it helpful when diagnosing the state of health and assessing the onset of any pathology.

COMPOSITION

The composition of interstitial lymph, also called *histolymph* or *intercellular fluid*, depends directly on the activity of the organs in which it is found. For example, in the case of an endocrine lymph node, the lymph will be very rich in hormones produced by that gland. It is like an underground stream whose composition depends on the terrain through which it flows.

In general, the composition of lymph is very similar to that of blood plasma, although it differs in the proportion of proteins, which is almost halved in this case. Lymph coagulates on contact with air, probably because it contains those coagulating substances that are also found in blood. The amount of proteins present in lymph varies from one area of the body to another. For example, lymph of hepatic origin is 6.6% protein, while that of cutaneous origin is only 2% protein.

As mentioned above, lymph contains some of the many substances derived from cellular metabolism: enzymes, hormones, metabolic residues, and traces of other compounds, as well as a small number of red blood cells and lymphocytes.

Some elements and compounds are found in a constant percentage.

VOLUME

The volume of histolymph can be calculated by subtracting the volume of fluid carried into the tissue by the arterial capillary from the volume of fluid reabsorbed at the other end by the venous capillary.

Mineral Content and Main Compounds in Plasma, Histolymph, and Intracellular Fluids

Element	Plasma	Histolymph	Intracellular Fluids
Na (sodium)	127–142	127–148	30
K (potassium)	4	4	118
Mg (magnesium)	2	2	30
Ca (calcium)	4–5	3–4.7	5
HCO_3 (bicarbonate)	27	32	10
Cl (chlorine)	96–104	98–114	28
HPO_4 (hydrogen phosphate)	2	2	80
Sulphate	trace	1	22
Organic acids	1	1	trace
Protein binding	26	2	50
Protein (g/100 ml)	7	2.8–4.89	155

Apart from protein, whose values are expressed in g/100 ml, all other data are expressed in milliequivalents per liter (mEq/l). The chemical equivalent, or equivalent weight, is the amount in grams of each chemical element expressed with the same number as the atomic weight; the milliequivalent (mEq) is one-thousandth of the equivalent.

In a sense, the histolymph and the intercellular space it occupies act as a buffer vessel through the exchange of fluids between the arterial and venous sections of the tissue.

If the arterial capillary leaves a larger amount of fluid, it is collected in the space occupied by the histolymph and is gradually released into the venous capillary to avoid too-rapid emptying. Excess fluid is absorbed by the lymphatic capillary and then is conducted into the lymphatic vessels.

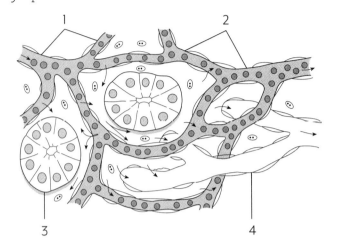

Lymphatic capillaries of a lymph node (consisting of many glandular grains) in relation to venous and arterial capillaries. The arrows indicate the direction of the lymph.

1. Arterial capillaries
2. Venous capillaries
3. Glandular grain
4. Lymphatic capillary

Conversely, if arterial flow is reduced, then histolymph leaves fluids in the venous capillary to prevent collapse of the walls due to a vacuum.

Each day, the histolymph collects two to four liters of fluid, which is put back into circulation.

HISTOLYMPH FORMATION FROM CAPILLARY CIRCULATION

Two factors are related to the formation: homeostasis (balanced maintenance) and the eventual pathology of the histolymph:

- vascular hydrodynamic pressure;
- osmotic pressure.

The vascular hydrodynamic pressure is that pressure in the capillary vessel that pushes the plasma outward, i.e., toward the cell and the histolymph in which the cells are immersed. It is derived from cardiac buoyancy, meaning the activity of the muscle in which the vessel is located and the elasticity of the vessel wall itself.

Osmotic pressure ("osmotic" coming from the Greek word *osmos*, which could be translated as "push" or "impulse") is generated between two compartments containing solutions of different concentrations, separated by a semipermeable membrane (which allows the liquid or solvent and, partially, the dissolved substance or solute to pass through). The solvent, whose task is to establish the equilibrium of the solute concentration, passes from the solution whose concentration is lower to the one with the higher concentration. In the separation membrane, this flow exerts a force called *osmotic pressure*.

All cell membranes, as well as those of the cells of the inner wall (endothelium) of capillaries, are semipermeable membranes that separate the capillary compartment from the histolymph. The solute, in this case, consists of proteins with a molecular weight of more than 5,000 (when the molecular weight is lower, the proteins spread freely in the solvent; however, although in small proportions and very slowly, even albumin proteins with a high molecular weight, up to 70,000, manage to overcome the endothelial membrane). The solute also contains blood cells, which are numerous in this medium but not in the histolymph.

THE PRESSURE

In physics, pressure is the ratio of a force acting perpendicular to a surface to the area of the same surface.

The official unit of measurement is the newton[1] (N) per square meter, called pascal (Pa) after the French physicist Blaise Pascal (1623–1662), who conducted several studies on the pressure of gases. Other units of measurement are also used, such as the bar (and especially its thousandth fraction, the millibar), which are used in meteorology: 1 bar corresponds to 100,000 pascals or 0.986 atmospheres. The atmosphere (Atm), in turn, is the atmospheric pressure

---

1   The newton (N) is the unit of measure for force and is equal to the mass of 1 kg multiplied by the acceleration of 1 m per second.

at sea level, equivalent to 760 Torr, i.e., the pressure exerted by a column of mercury with a cross-section of one square centimeter and a height of 760 mm. The millimeter of mercury (mm Hg) is also called Torr, after the Italian physicist Evangelista Torricelli (1608–1647), a disciple of Galileo and inventor of the mercury barometer.

There are other units of measurement for pressure, although in medicine the measurement in millimeters of mercury is used.

As shown in the table on page 9, the protein concentration in histolymph is about half that found in blood, or rather plasma (7 g/100 ml in plasma and 3.5 g/100 ml in histolymph), with very wide variations from one tissue to another, which is why the osmotic pressure is also not the same in all capillary zones.

Due to the variability of proteins in the histolymph, an average pressure (called *oncotic*) is established, which depends on the contained elements that tend to push against the current (e.g. in the histolymph of the digestive tract just after digestion), toward the inside of the capillaries. This phenomenon is considered in the following table.

Pressure	Capillary Type	Capillary Arteriovenous	Capillary
Outward from the capillary	Vascular hydrostatic	32 mm Hg	18 mm Hg
Outside the capillary	Osmotic histolymph	5 mm Hg	5 mm Hg
Inward from the capillary	Histolymph hydrostatic	5 mm Hg (0–10)	5 mm Hg (0–10)
Inward plasma	Osmotic capillary	25 mm Hg	25 mm Hg

Total outward pressure = vascular hydrostatic + histolymph osmotic:

Arterial: 32 + 5 = 37 mm Hg

Venous: 18 + 5 = 23 mm Hg

Total inward pressure = histolymph hydrostatic + plasma osmotic:

Arterial: 5 + 25 = 30 mm Hg

Venous: 5 + 25 = 30 mm Hg

Total pressure difference = total outward pressure–total inward pressure:

Arterial: 37–30 = 7 mm Hg

Venous: 23–30 = 7 mm Hg

This pressure difference between the outflow of the arterial capillary and the inflow of the venous capillary allows the physiological exchange of histolymph and microcirculation. The balance can be disturbed in different cases, which relate to two main problems:

- decrease in osmotic pressure within the venous capillary due to lack of protein in the blood;
- increased hydrostatic pressure in the veins.

The lack of protein, in turn, is due to one of three main factors:

- kidney disease: when the kidney fails to retain protein, it is eliminated through the urine, causing a drastic reduction in the osmotic pressure of the histolymph, which allows fluid resorption;
- defects in intestinal resorption, as in celiac morbidity;
- liver diseases or situations of prolonged prostration after acute illnesses or due to chronic diseases or intensive drug treatments. This results in insufficient protein synthesis by the liver.

The increase in venous hydrostatic pressure occurs when the upright position is maintained for a long time, without muscular movement, as occurs in the case of all those persons who remain standing for a large part of the day. The venous pressure in the capillary circuit of the legs can reach 90 mm Hg, causing stagnation of the histolymph and consequent swelling, especially in the ankles; if this situation continues, venous insufficiency can occur.

Venous hydrostatic pressure may be increased as a result of an obstruction in deflux caused by inflammation or tumor masses.

CIRCULATING LYMPH

PERIPHERAL LYMPH AND LYMPHATIC CAPILLARIES

Peripheral lymph can be compared to spring water containing traces of the minerals that make up the rocks from which it emerges. In our case, the source of the lymphatic circulation is histolymph (see the chapter on the *grundsystem*, page 17).

Just as it can be said that there is a relationship between the active force of the sun and the passive force of the earth—which receives water from the atmosphere and returns it purified and ready for a new life cycle—so in mankind, the active part of the system is the heart while the passive part is the histolymph. Moreover, the heart is almost centrally located within the body, while the histolymph circulates throughout the body. Based on these statements, the histolymph could be considered a "peripheral pump" of the lymphatic circulation.

Peripheral lymph contains traces of the chemical composition and production of the tissue from which it originates. It contains little more protein than histolymph and few lymph cells.

Lymphatic capillaries, through which peripheral lymph passes, are difficult to identify in tissue analysis (histological sections). Therefore, even in those tissues where they do not seem to exist (bone marrow, lung alveoli, cartilage, epithelia, fetal placenta, spleen pulp, and central nervous system), some form of lymphatic activity cannot be completely excluded.

In contrast, there is a dense lymphatic network in the dermis, as well as in the periosteum (a thin membrane with many nerves surrounding the bones) and also in the submucosa of the digestive, genital, urinary, and respiratory organs.

Lymphatic capillaries emerging from the intercellular space range in diameter from 10 to 40 microns (twice the diameter of an average-sized capillary) and are highly irregular in shape and caliber.

The walls of capillaries and lymphatic vessels are composed of larger but thinner endothelial cells[2] than the endothelium of venous vessels. In addition, the space between them is larger in lymphatic vessels than in blood vessels, allowing communication and exchange between both circulating and interstitial lymph. This space is particularly wide in the lymphatic vessels of the diaphragm and is filled with a fluid that is extremely rich in water.

In the lymphatic capillaries, finally, the basement membrane (the equivalent of the impermeable substances that are placed under the soil of the "terraces") is missing, though it is present in an increasingly clear and continuous manner in the larger lymphatic vessels, where muscle cells are also gathered around them.

THE INTERMEDIATE LYMPH

The intermediate lymph circulates in larger lymphatic vessels, whose wall thickness resembles the wall of smaller veins.

It contains numerous lymphocytes originating from the lymph nodes, or the main production centers for such cells.

THE CENTRAL LYMPH

The central lymph circulates in large lymphatic ducts (see the chapter on lymphatic circulation, page 25).

Approximately five *trillion* lymphocytes are introduced or reintroduced into the blood each day through the thoracic duct; in fact, the number of new white blood cells represents only a small percentage of those carried in the blood through that duct.

---

2 The endothelium, i.e., the tissue that lines the inside of vessels, is very similar to a tiled floor, the tiles of which would be the cells.

Chapter 2

THE BASIC SYSTEM OR GRUNDSYSTEM

THE CELL

The cell is the basic unit of living organisms and has an autonomous life. It consists of a membrane that separates it from the outside world and through which the cell takes in the oxygen and food it needs both to live and to eliminate waste substances. It also has a sensory function (like our five human senses) and can distinguish toxic substances from useful ones.

Inside the cell is a complex structure, called the *endoplasmic reticulum*, which performs a function similar to that of the intestine and is used by the cell to expel waste and produce certain substances, such as enzymes in the case of the pancreatic cell.

There are also cylindrical or ovoid structures, called *mitochondria*, which resemble microscopic "boilers" and use oxygen to burn food fuel to produce energy.

Roughly in the center of the cell, in the most protected place, is the nucleus. This is where the DNA is found—a large, helix-shaped structure in which the individual genetic code is encoded.

As has been pointed out, a cell is able to live autonomously and in the company of many others, as is the case in humans. In this way, cells find a better system to ensure their survival and enable their own activity.

THE *GRUNDSYSTEM*

WHAT IS THE *GRUNDSYSTEM*?

The basic system, also called *grundsystem*, according to Pischinger's definition, consists of the smallest cellular community that can be found within a tissue, such as, in human society, a village or a neighborhood of a city.

Cells are the individuals that make up the organism and that, by coming together and specializing according to anatomical and functional characteristics, form a "nation," i.e., an organism. Within this organism, therefore, various types of tissue (nervous, skeletal, muscular, connective, cartilaginous, lymphatic, hematic, and others) are differentiated.

The concept of *grundsystem* refers to the smallest organizational unit within the tissue, which in turn is found within the organism.

FROM THE GRUNDSYSTEM TO THE LYMPHATIC SYSTEM

Each organ, therefore, is made up of different types of tissue, and each tissue contains several thousand intercellular units, which we have called *grundsystem*, resembling tiny lymph nodes (see pages 49–53). From these originate lymphatic capillaries, which run inside the organ, constituting its own particular system, practically parallel to the venous system.

Smaller lymph nodes may belong to the organ's lymphatic system, interposed along the path of the lymphatic capillaries inside the organ, whose function is to filter the incoming lymph, enriching it if necessary, with antibodies or cells for immune defense (called immunocompetent cells).

The lymphatic capillaries subsequently join together to form larger trunks, which carry the lymph to the outside of the organ. Close to the outer wall are a number of lymph nodes, which also serve to filter and immunologically defend the lymph.

PLASMA FLOW IN THE *GRUNDSYSTEM*

The cells are immersed in intercellular fluid, or histolymph, derived from blood plasma (the liquid part of the blood) that reaches the *grundsystem* through an arterial capillary.

The plasma coming from the small artery transports oxygen and nourishment to the cells; these, dissolved in the intercellular fluid, are absorbed by each cell according to its needs.

Subsequently, the cell, after being nourished and obtaining the energy it needs to live and carry out its functions, expels the waste, depositing it in the intercellular fluid stream that flows into a vein.

The histolymph thus moves by means of a current, in the same way as water flows into a lake in a tributary and out through an underground channel.

If we were to represent the lymphatic system as a lake, the tributary would consist precisely of the arterial capillary that carries the plasma. This, in the *grundsystem*, becomes intercellular fluid.

The canal, by contrast, has a dual function: there is a small, thinner tube, whose current runs faster, called the *venous capillary*, capable of transporting dissolved gases and in particular carbon dioxide, which must be transported rapidly to the lungs to be expelled and exchanged for oxygen. There is also a second, wider tube, whose current runs slower, called the *lymphatic capillary*.

The lymphatic capillary can collect and remove coarser residual particles, such as bacteria and other heavier substances, from the *grundsystem*. It is also a reserve reservoir, a kind of compensation vessel in cases where the venous capillary, for the reasons explained in the first chapter, is unable to remove fluids. These liquids would in fact swell the *grundsystem* excessively, even endangering the life of the cells present in it. The lymphatic capillary therefore performs the functions of a real drainage channel.

GRUNDSYSTEM PATHOLOGIES

In relation to what has been stated above, *grundsystem* disturbance can be mainly due to any of five causes that are at the basis of any pathology. Therapy is aimed at curing one or more of these causes.

THE FIVE CAUSES OF DISEASE

1. **Defective flow through the arterial capillary:** this can originate in arteriosclerosis or in Reynaud's syndrome, in which there is a spasm of the smooth muscle of the small artery, whose caliber decreases.

2. **Irregular uptake of nutrients by the cell:** this may be due to a defect in the cell membrane or to a lack of insulin (which carries sugar molecules into the cell) or even to chemical mediators (substances that stimulate the cell's uptake activity).

3. **Problems in the elimination of waste products by the cell:** these are caused by viral diseases, contamination, intoxication, and other causes.

4. **Difficult expulsion of *grundsystem* residues through the venous system:** this may be due to thrombosis, trauma, compression, increased venous hydrostatic pressure (with consequent venous insufficiency), or protein deficiencies due to renal, intestinal, hepatic, and metabolic diseases that increase the venous osmotic pressure toward the histolymph.

5. **Problems in the elimination of waste through the lymphatic capillary:** these may be due to trauma, compression, infection, contamination, and others.

These five causes mainly influence the circulation of lymph through the interior of each organ. This means that a lymphatic stasis dependent on an organ dysfunction can lead to a further worsening of the organ dysfunction (if it is not its initial cause) as well as to other disorders and diseases.

For example, lymphatic stasis in the heart leads to rhythm dysfunctions and infarction; in the kidney, it can lead to a greater or lesser degree of kidney failure, increased blood pressure, and even anemia; in the bronchi and lungs, it causes or prolongs respiratory problems and defective breathing and oxygenation of the blood, as in chronic bronchitis or allergic asthma; in skeletal muscle, it often leads to muscle stiffness and loss of elasticity, with consequent ease of muscle and tendon strain, ligament sprain, and joint distress, greatly reducing mobility.

By contrast, lymphatic stasis in an organ can be made more serious by excessive fatigue, trauma, intoxication, or infections caused by fungi, bacteria, viruses, and the like. It can also be caused by the disease of a nearby organ blocking the lymphatic outflow pathways, or by the presence of obstacles in the path of the total or partial circulation of lymph.

THE DIAGNOSIS

The lymphatic system, and in particular the lymphatic system of each organ, is one of an organism's functional groups that is most sensitive to disease.

How can lymphatic stasis of an organ be diagnosed?

In principle, organ dysfunction can often be identified through the patient's medical history, especially when it begins shortly after a period of fatigue, trauma, intoxication, or bacterial, viral, or fungal infection. Subsequently, more specific examinations must be carried out. One of the main ones is the electrical measurement of certain acupuncture points, called *lymphatic points*, according to Dr. Reinhold Voll's EAV (see page 186). That system is convenient, has no side effects, and is undoubtedly highly effective, as it makes it possible to establish by measuring specific points the loss of function of each part of the body's lymphatic system and then to determine its causes.

The EAV is therefore a privileged method in disease prevention, as it can detect disorders in the organism at an early stage. In addition, it makes it possible to find out precisely and quickly which therapy is needed to restore balance and prevent a worsening of the pathology, which could progress from simple dysfunction even to anatomical alteration.

THE PHASES OF THE DISEASE

According to German physician H. H. Reckeweg, the founder of homotoxicology (according to which it is possible to purify and regenerate the organism by means of homeopathic products), illness is *not* a random and unforeseen event, but instead results from the progressive intoxication of the *grundsystem* through six specific phases:

1. **Excretion:** the lymphatic flow increases in order to discharge toxins that are poured in excess into the histolymph. Symptoms are those of an acute cold that disappears in a short time, increased lacrimation, increased bowel movement or breathing, painful elimination of urine, and other symptoms.

2. **Inflammation:** the body produces substances that call for blood in a certain part of the body, resulting in an increased flow of white blood cells. This occurs when the physiological excretion is not sufficient to remove the toxins from the histolymph of the

grundsystem. Symptoms are redness, swelling, heat, pain, and a functional disturbance of the tissue. Inflammation is typical in acute diseases with a more violent course, when the *grundsystem* is endowed with good defenses.

3. **Deposition:** toxins accumulate in the histolymph. This occurs when the body is unable to expel the toxins completely either by normal means or through increased local circulation, as in the case of inflammation. This can lead to the formation of kidney stones, gallstones, skin blemishes, osteoarthritis, and so on.

4. **Impregnation:** toxins enter the cells, alter their functionality, and damage them. It occurs in long-term viral illnesses and prolonged intoxication due to smoke and pollution. The general symptoms are profound fatigue, depression, memory and movement coordination disorders, and the like.

5. **Degeneration:** the cell damaged by toxins is unable to carry out its normal functions. This is the case, for example, in polio, multiple sclerosis, arteriosclerosis, and autoimmune diseases.

6. **Assimilation:** the toxins attack the cell's DNA, which loses its own genetic code, causing its relationship with the organism to disappear. This is the phase in which tumors and diseases such as schizophrenia develop.

However, it should be remembered that there are several tissues in an organism, so its *grundsystem* can therefore be at different stages of disease.

THERAPY AND HEALING

The maintenance or restoration of health is possible through a number of fundamental practices that can significantly influence the *grundsystem*. These practices are the following:

- food;
- physical exercise;

- meditation or relaxation and concentration practices;
- lymphatic drainage;
- homeopathy and homotoxicology (see pages 201–206);
- acupuncture;
- general health practices: massages, rubbing compresses, and the like.

Often, during the healing process, there is what in homeopathy is called a *worsening*, i.e., a worsening of the symptoms prior to their extinction. This happens because the disease, in its process, goes through the different phases. For example, if a sick person is in the deposition phase, in order to be cured he or she will have to go through the inflammatory phase and then the excretion phase.

With appropriate therapeutic measures, this worsening of symptoms can be minimized and rendered harmless, without hindering the normal elimination of toxins.

From the fourth stage (impregnation), full functional recovery is difficult, if not impossible. The disease, however, if treated promptly, does not worsen and sometimes even regresses.

Chapter 3

LYMPH CIRCULATION
Microcirculation and Lymphatic Vessels

The previous chapters have discussed the general characteristics of the lymph and the *grundsystem*. It has also been pointed out how lymph drainage is one of the practices that can positively influence the basic system. Now, before going into the part on techniques for effective lymph drainage, it is necessary to clarify some topics about the functioning and anatomy of the lymphatic system (for an overview of the lymphatic circulation, see pages 69–70).

MICROCIRCULATION

Microcirculation is the system made up of tiny arterial, venous, and lymphatic vessels with a caliber of less than 20 microns (one micron is one thousandth of a millimeter).

The density of the microcirculation varies from one tissue to another. It is absent, for example, in some cartilage, in the crystalline lens, and in the intervertebral discs of people over 20 years of age. In muscle, the density of microcirculation increases from five capillaries per square millimeter in resting tissue to 190 capillaries in moving muscle, thus increasing 40-fold from one phase to the next. In brain, on the other hand, the number of open capillaries remains constant, as the nerve cell, lacking a reserve of extracellular fluid, needs constant nourishment.

The mean pressure in the arteries is 90 mm Hg (see pages 10–14); as the vascular caliber shrinks, the pressure decreases and is partially transformed into heat due to the friction of the blood on the vascular walls. Hydraulic resistance, which is inversely proportional to the vessel radius raised to the fourth power, increases markedly at the capillary level, to the point where the mean pressure drops to 35 mm Hg. About 60 mm Hg is thus transformed into heat, which is why microcirculation is the most important system for heating the body, based on the friction of blood and lymph on the vascular walls.

In the capillaries, blood circulates at an average speed of 70 microns per second, about 500 times slower than in the aorta. This allows for the exchange of oxygen, carbon dioxide, nutrients (anabolites), and waste substances (catabolites). This exchange occurs either directly between blood and cells (in tissues such as the nervous and pulmonary alveoli, in which histolymph appears to be absent) or between histolymph and blood through the capillary wall, which is about 1 micron thick. The length of the capillary network, from the beginning of the arterial capillary to the end of the venous capillary, ranges from 400 to 700 microns.

In humans, the total surface area of the capillary walls in muscle tissue alone, which constitutes 40% of the total body mass, has been estimated at over 64,000 square feet; in the whole organism, therefore, the capillary surface area available for gaseous, nutritional, and depurative exchanges is at least 107,000 square feet.

LYMPHATIC CAPILLARIES

Lymphatic capillaries consist of an inner layer (endothelium) and a thin porous membrane. The endothelium is made up of attached cells that have a smooth surface and allow better lymph circulation. In contrast, the outer membrane is porous and enables the lymphatic capillaries to absorb intercellular fluids from the tissues they pass through.

When the tissue is inflamed and swollen, the pores open to evacuate excess fluids.

The increasingly larger vessels into which the lymphatic capillaries converge are much thinner than the corresponding venous vessels.

FROM LYMPHATIC CAPILLARIES TO LYMPHATIC DUCTS

From the *grundsystem*, therefore, a complex network is built of initially very small vessels, the lymphatic capillaries, which are mostly located inside the organs and tissues drained by them.

The capillaries, in turn, converge in small lymphatic vessels, often close to the organ wall or the outer surface of the tissue.

The lymph therefore passes through the small-caliber lymphatic vessels and then through the medium-caliber vessels, which in turn collect the lymph from the other adjacent organs and tissues.

The lymphatic trunks, also called lymphatic ducts or terminal trunks, are formed from the confluence of the medium-caliber lymphatic vessels (for their location, see the figure on page 29). They are as follows:

- thoracic duct: the largest lymphatic duct;
- subclavian duct, right and left;
- jugular duct, right and left;
- bronchomediastinal trunk, right and left;
- intestinal tract or duct;

- large right lymphatic vein: this is a supplementary trunk, not always present, that collects lymph from the right chest wall, which usually flows into the thoracic duct;
- Pecquet's cistern or duct[3]: this is highly variable in shape and dimensions.

For the position of the terminal trunks, see the figure on page 29. In addition to the thoracic duct, the other lymphatic trunks or ducts also join in the hematic system between the subclavian vein and the jugular vein, and may arrive alone or otherwise converge with each other.

Depending on its origin, there are two types of lymph:
- visceral lymph, which comes from the internal organs;
- parietal lymph, which comes from the extremities (as in walls of the face, thorax, abdomen, muscles, and supporting tissues) and is further differentiated into both deep parietal lymph, which derives from the deeper muscle and supporting struc- tures, and superficial parietal lymph, which derives from the subcutis and superficial muscle layers.

Manual lymphatic drainage, although it mainly affects the superficial parietal lymphatic circulation (see pages 81–153), achieves some effect even on the deep parietal and visceral lymph. This may occur because the sectors of the lymphatic system are mutually related.

THE LYMPHATIC VESSELS

The lymphatic vessels, seen externally, look like the shells of legumes: in fact, their diameter is not uniform, but they have swellings at regular distances that correspond to valves that prevent the lymph from flowing backwards. In relation to the lymphatic capillaries, the

---

3   It is named after the French physician Jean Pecquet (1622–1674), who described it together with the thoracic duct in his *Experimenta Anatomica* (1651).

vessels have a structure similar to that of small veins; they are up to 1 mm thick and have a dense network of muscle fibers, coiled in a spiral around the vessel. The lymphatic vessels can push the lymph along its course.

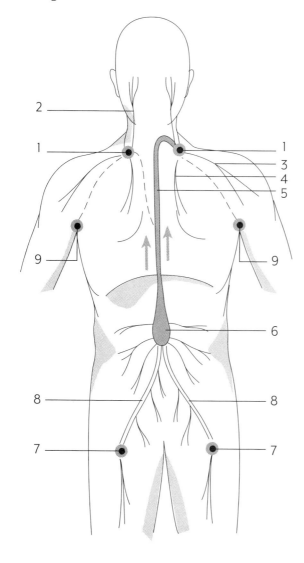

Diagram of the main ducts of the lymphatic circulation. The position of the inguinal lymph nodes and the iliac lymphatic vessels, which must be taken into account in the treatment of cellulitis, is also indicated (see pages 132–137 and 170–173).

1. Terminus
2. Jugular duct
3. Subclavian duct
4. Broncho-diastinal duct
5. Thoracic duct
6. Pecquet's cistern
7. Inguinal lymph nodes
8. Iliac lymphatic vessels
9. Axillary lymph nodes

LYMPH CIRCULATION

How does lymph make its way through the lymphatic vessels? There are six main factors:

1. The contraction of the muscles in which the lymphatic vessels are located: when compressed, they push the lymph in one direction only, as the valves prevent its reflux.
2. The thin, loosely packed musculature around the larger vessels, arranged in a spiral, helps to regulate the circulation of lymph (normally there is a contraction of the vessel musculature every two breaths).
3. A kind of whirlwind, caused by the thoracic duct on the lymph during the inspiration phase, moves the lymph toward the thorax.
4. Arterial pulsations close to the lymphatic vessels press on the outer wall of these vessels and push the lymph.
5. The pressure exerted on the lymphatic and venous vessels of the sole of the foot, during habitual movements, pushes the lymph. If a person stands upright for a long time, this push, which is essential for the lymphatic and venous circulation of the leg, will be impeded. By contrast, the lack of contraction of the muscles will not be able to push the lymph and, consequently, the whole process will be affected; this is why it is easier for the ankles to be swollen in the evening and the foot and leg to feel heavy.
6. The heartbeat, which pushes on the thoracic duct, is also involved in the circulation.

THE LYMPHATIC PATHWAY

The lymph moves mainly in the direction opposite to the force of gravity, thanks to the valves and pushing mechanisms described above. In the head and neck, though, the opposite is true, as the drained lymph is directed upwards and downward to the lymph nodes below the clavicle, which are also known as the *terminus* (see page 29).

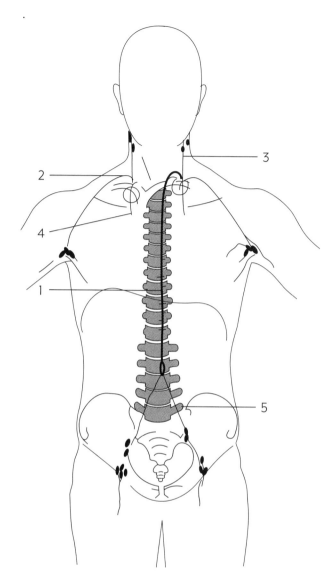

The main lymphatic ducts with their drained territory

1. Thoracic duct (starts at Pecquet's cistern). Parietal lymph: leg, abdomen, thorax. Visceral lymph: part of the thorax and abdomen, excluding the liver.

2. Subclavian duct. Parietal lymph: arms.

3. Jugular duct. Parietal and visceral lymph: head and neck.

4. Bronchomediastinal duct. Visceral lymph: organs of the thorax (heart and lungs) and liver.

5. Intestinal tract (reaches Pecquet's cistern). Visceral lymph: organs of the abdomen, excluding the liver.

LEGS

The lymph coming from the sole of the foot and the back of the leg goes to the lymph nodes at the back of the knee; from there it follows the route of the large deep venous vessels to the inguinal lymph nodes and from there to the inside of the pelvis. Some of the problems with lymphatic circulation at this level are caused by incorrect posture, especially when one is in an upright position, but also in a sitting position. The edge of a chair, in fact, by compressing the back of the thigh, slows down the lymphatic and venous flow to the pelvis, which facilitates the formation of cellulite in the knee and thighs. To avoid this problem, reclining stools can be used that elevate the legs and thus prevent excessive compression of the back of the thigh and at the same time force the spine into a more natural, uncurved position. Lymph from the instep of the foot, the anterior surface of the leg and the thigh goes to the inguinal lymph nodes and from there to the inner part of the pelvis.

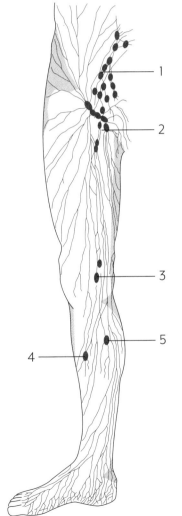

Lymphatic circulation of the leg

1. Deep inguinal lymph nodes
2. Superficial inguinal lymph nodes
3. Popliteal lymph nodes (from the back of the knee)
4. Anterior tibial lymph node
5. Posterior tibial lymph node

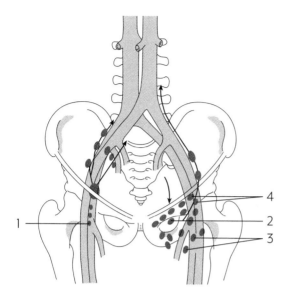

The four groups of inguinal lymph nodes (upper external and internal, lower external and internal) with their respective drainage areas

1. Deep lymph of the lower extremities

2. Abdominal wall, external genitalia, and perineum

3. Superficial circle of the leg

4. Abdominal wall and buttocks

THE PELVIS

Part of the lymph coming from the sacral region (the ischium is the bony part of the pelvis on which we lean when sitting), from the perineal region (the anal and genital areas), and from the upper and inner thighs close to the perineum goes to the lower inguinal lymph nodes. Another part enters directly into the pelvis, along the genital organs and rectum. Therefore, if a woman has cellulitis, especially in the upper and inner thighs, she is likely to suffer from infections of the genital organs as well as from constipation and hemorrhoids. Men are less prone to cellulite than women, but they can experience some pathologies, such as prostatic hyper dystrophy or repeated prostate inflammation, constipation, and hemorrhoids, which in turn can lead to lymphatic stasis. The median line of the thighs forms a sort of watershed between the lymphatic vessels that run to the inguinal lymph nodes, following a path from the inside to the outside, and that carry them to the inguinal lymph nodes through the inner thighs. The lymphatic vessels of the buttocks, except those of the sacral region, go in the direction of the inguinal lymph nodes, circling the thigh from the inside to the outside and from the back to the front.

THE ABDOMEN

Lymph from the abdominal wall below the waistline is directed toward the inguinal lymph nodes.

The lymphatic vessels of the abdominal organs and from most of the lower abdominal wall, as well as from the urogenital organs, rectum, buttocks, and legs, converge through the intestinal and lumbar ducts into Pecquet's cistern, which is variable in shape and lies in front of the spinal column, approximately at the level of the second lumbar vertebra, is about 2 cm long and 1 cm or more wide, where the thoracic duct originates.

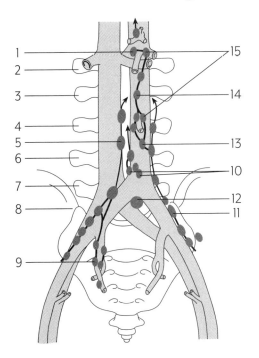

1. Stomach and bile ducts
2. First lumbar vertebra
3. Second lumbar vertebra
4. Third lumbar vertebra
5. Right lumbar trunk to Pecquet's cistern
6. Fourth lumbar vertebra
7. Fifth lumbar vertebra
8. Leg and pelvic walls
9. Internal iliac lymph nodes
10. Viscera and pelvis
11. Lateral common iliac lymph nodes
12. Promontory lymph nodes
13. Left lumbar trunk to Pecquet's cistern
14. Pecquet's cistern
15. Small intestine and pelvic colon

The sacrolumbar lymphatic circulation is made possible by lymph nodes around the abdominal aorta. Note that there are some lymphatic tributaries arising from the different territories of the abdomen.

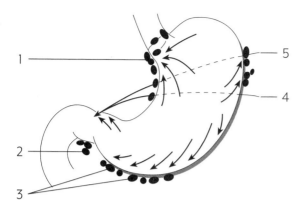

Lymphatic circulation of
the stomach and adjoining
lymph nodes

1. Upper gastric lymph nodes
2. Subpyloric station
3. Lower gastric lymph nodes
4. Pancreas
5. Spleen

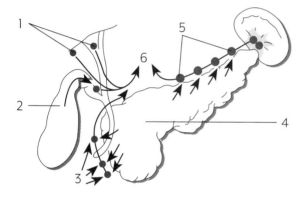

*Lymphatic circulation of the
pancreas*

1. Hepatic lymph nodes
2. Gallbladder
3. Pancreatic and duodenal
lymph nodes
4. Pancreas
5. Lienal and pancreatic
lymph nodes
6. Retropyloric station

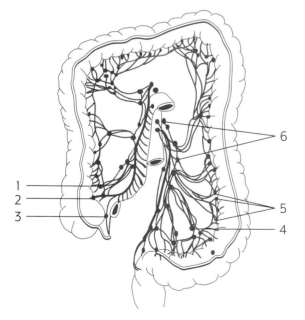

*Lymphatic circulation of the
large intestine*

1. Ileocolic lymph nodes
2. Blind lymph nodules
3. Appendicular lymph node
4. Intercolic lymph nodes
5. Paracolic lymph nodes
6. Lower mesenteric lymph
nodes

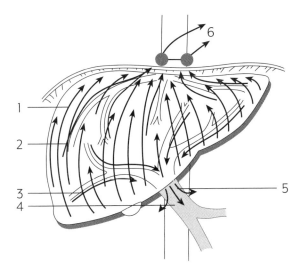

Lymphatic circulation of the liver

1. Superficial network (toward the coronary ligament)

2. Ascending lymphatic vessels (to the vena cava)

3. Descending lymphatic vessels (to the hepatic hilum)

4. Toward the retropyloric station

5. To the preaortic lymph nodes

6. Toward the mediastinal chains

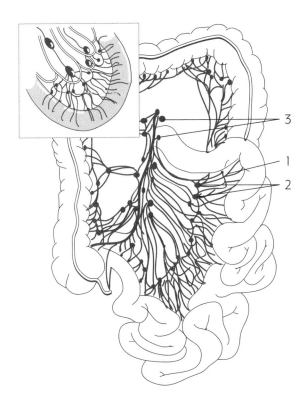

Lymphatic circulation of the small intestine. Note how lymph flows through three groups of lymph nodal stations, positioned close to the intestinal wall (1), in an intermediate position (2), and finally along the mesentery (3). The drawing shows a detail of the lymphatic vessels in an intestinal fold.

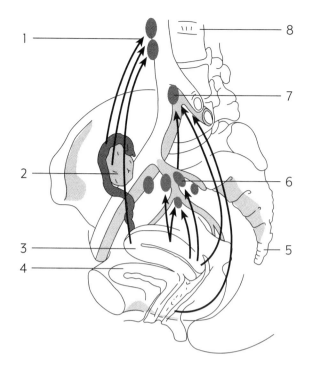

THE THORAX

From Pecquet's cistern starts the thoracic duct, which collects lymph from the abdominal organs, legs, hemithorax, left arm, and left side of the head. Going upward, after crossing the diaphragm, the thoracic duct moves to the left until it joins just below the clavicle, at the vein that collects venous blood from the left arm (the left subclavian vein).

On the right side of the thorax, parallel to the aorta, the large right lymphatic vein may glide, collecting lymph from the right hemithorax, the right arm, and the right side of the head, to finally reach, just below the clavicle, the right subclavian vein.

Lymph coming from the spine and the muscles closest to the spine enters directly into the left thoracic duct and sometimes also into the large right lymphatic vein.

Lymph from the deep back and thoracic musculature, the ribs, the intercostal muscles, and the cartilage of the thorax, goes to the intercostal lymphatic vessels, until it reaches the left thoracic duct and the large right lymphatic vein.

From the large superficial muscles of the thorax and spine (trapezius, latissimus dorsi, and pectoralis), from the upper part of the waist, from the breast and the subcutaneous tissue above it, the lymph passes, by contrast, following a superficial route, to the axillary lymph nodes; and from there, along the subclavian duct, it flows to the lymph nodes below the clavicle, to the left thoracic duct, to the large right lymphatic vein, or to the subclavian veins, near the junction between these and the veins of the neck.

Lymph from the heart, lungs, mediastinum (the space between heart, lungs, and great vessels), and liver is drained by the broncho-mediastinal trunk, which starts from the subclavian vein near the thoracic duct and enters the trunk before it ends.

For a diagram of the lymphatic circulation of the breast, see page 177.

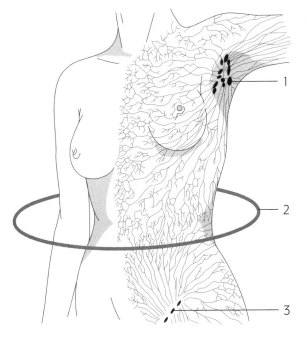

Superficial lymphatic circulation of the anterior part of the trunk

1. Toward the axillary lymph nodes

2. Separation between upper and lower trunk region

3. Inguinal lymph nodes

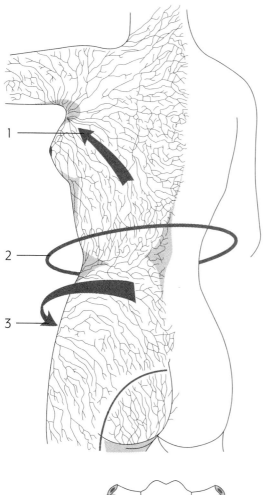

Superficial lymphatic circulation of the back of the trunk

1. To axillary lymph nodes
2. Separation between upper and lower trunk region
3. Toward the inguinal lymph nodes

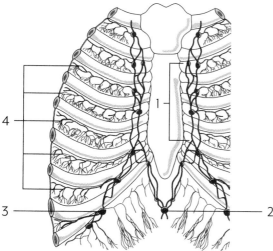

Lymphatic circulation in the anterior chest: note the position of the lymph nodes and the appearance of the intercostal lymphatic vessels.

1. Parasternal lymph nodes
2. Epigastric lymph nodes
3. Lymph nodes of the costal arch
4. Intercostal lymphatic circulation

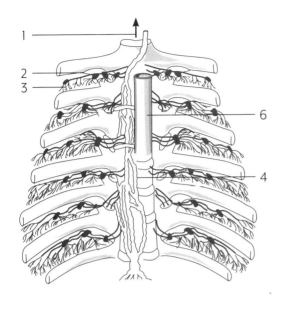

Lymphatic circulation in the posterior chest wall

1. Direction of lymphatic flow
2. Paravertebral lymph nodes
3. Intercostal lymph nodes
4. Thoracic duct
5. Pecquet's cistern
6. Thoracic aorta

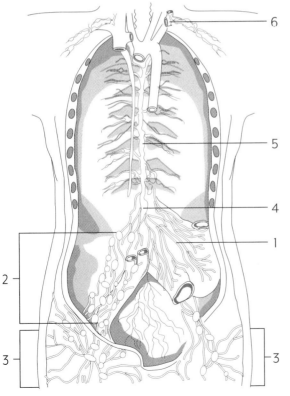

Distribution of the internal iliac lymph nodes and position of the thoracic duct. Note the relationship between the internal iliac and the inguinal lymph nodes. In addition, it can be seen how Pecquet's cistern also reaches the lymph from the internal organs of the abdomen.

1. Intestinal tract
2. Iliac vessels and lymph nodes
3. Inguinal lymph nodes
4. Pecquet's cistern
5. Thoracic duct
6. Thoracic duct opening into the left subclavian vein

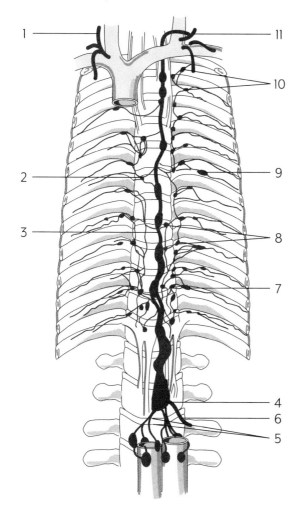

Origin and tributaries of the thoracic duct

1. Right jugular trunk
2. Spinal ganglion
3. Thoracic duct
4. Pecquet's cistern
5. Lumbar trunks (lymph from the walls of the abdomen and pelvis; visceral and limb lymph)
6. Intestinal trunk (intestinal visceral lymph)
7. Laterovertebral lymph nodules
8. Prevertebral lymph nodes
9. Intercostal lymph nodes
10. Ganglion of the first and second spaces
11. Left jugular trunk

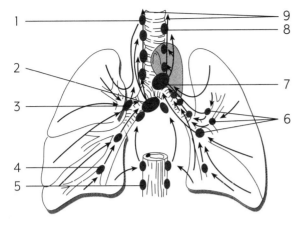

Lymphatic circulation of the airways and esophagus

1. Right laterotracheal lymph nodes

2. Lymph nodes of the bifurcation

3. Auxiliary stations

4. Right lung and deep right stations

5. Lymph nodes of the esophagus

6. Left deep lung stations

7. Pre-aortic lymph nodes

8. Left laterotracheal lymph nodules

9. Toward the bronchomediastinal trunk

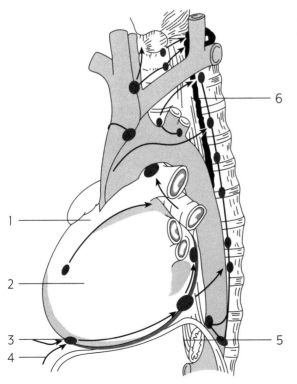

Lymphatic circulation of the heart

1. Toward the lymph nodes of the bifurcation

2. Heart

3. From the liver

4. From the diaphragm

5. Esophagus

6. Thoracic duct

THE ARMS

The lymphatic vessels of the arms carry lymph to the axillary lymph nodes, from which the subclavian duct originates, which then branches off to the right and left subclavian veins.

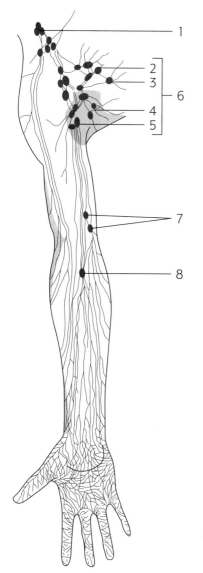

Lymphatic circulation and lymph nodes of the arm

1. Lymph nodes superior and inferior to the clavicle
2. Subpectoral lymph nodes
3. Intermediate lymph nodes
4. Inferior scapular lymph nodes
5. Brachial lymph nodes
6. Superficial and deep axillary lymph nodes
7. Cubital lymph nodes
8. Deep cubital lymph nodes

THE HEAD

The lymphatic vessels of the face roughly follow the three branches of the trigeminal, which constitute the innervation of the face.

From the upper part of the face, the lymph reaches the parotid lymph nodes in front of the ear. From there, following the anterior lateral part of the neck, it travels down to the lymph nodes below the scapula, flowing into the right or left subclavian vein or into the thoracic duct.

The lymphatic vessels of the midface are directed toward the angulus lymph nodes, so called because they are located in the angle of the jaw. From here the route is the same as that of the parotid lymph nodes.

From the lower face, the lymph goes to the lymph nodes near the submaxillary salivary nodes and then to the lymph nodes under the scapula.

The lymphatic vessels of the forehead reach the parotid lymph nodes. Those vessels of the temples reach the lymph nodes behind the ear, also called *mastoid*, as they are situated very close to or above the mastoid. The lymphatic vessels from the back of the skull join the lymph nodes of the shoulder blade.

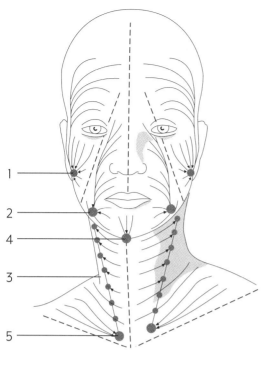

Anterior lymphatic circulation of the face and neck. The dashed lines separate the parotid and submaxillary lymph node regions according to their areas of competence. The anterior neck chains collect lymph from the two specular halves of the neck.

1. Lymph nodes earphones

2. Submaxillary lymph nodes

3. Latero-anterior lymph nodes of the neck

4. Chin lymph nodes

5. Terminus

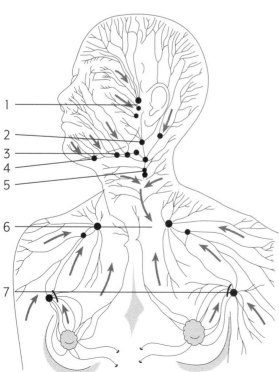

Schematic representation of the lymphatic circulation of the head, neck, and upper thorax. Note the confluence of the lymph, coming from the different regions, at the end of the lymphatic circulation.

1. Auricular or parotid lymph nodes

2. Inferior auricular lymph nodes (profundus)

3. Submaxillary lymph nodes

4. Chin lymph nodes

5. Laterocervical lymph nodes

6. Terminus (mouth of the main lymphatic ducts into the subclavian vein)

7. Axillary lymph nodes

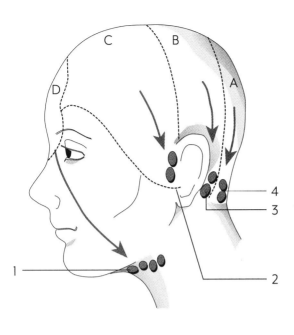

Lymphatic circulation of the cranial vault and the scalp

A. Direction of lymph from the occipital area

B. Direction of lymph from the parietal region

C. Direction of lymph from the parietotemporal region

D. Direction of lymph from the frontal region

1. Submaxillary lymph nodes

2. Anterior auricular or parotid lymph nodes

3. Posterior auricular lymph nodes

4. Occipital lymph nodes

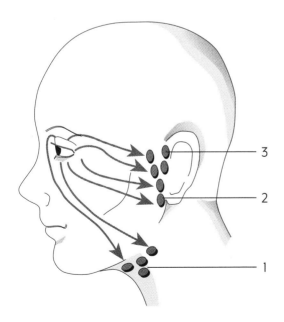

Lymphatic circulation of the eye and orbital region

1. Submaxillary lymph nodes

2. Anteroinferior auricular lymph nodes

3. Anterior auricular or parotid lymph nodes

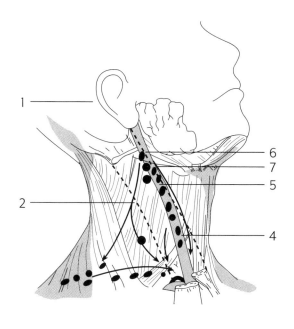

Anterolateral deep lymphatic circulation of the neck

1. Occipital region
2. Column chain
3. Transverse jugular chain
4. Internal jugular chain
5. Lateral and retropharyngeal region
6. Parotid region
7. Deep regions of the face

From the parotid lymph nodes, as mentioned above, and also from those behind the ear and the cervix, some lymphatic vessels arise that reach the lymph nodes below the scapula and from there go to the left thoracic duct and the large right lymphatic vein.

THE SHOULDERS

The lymph coming from the region at the level of the shoulder line, also called the *upper trapezius region* (in fact it has the shape of a layer whose lower vertex is located at the level of the seventh cervical vertebra),[4] reaches the lymph nodes below the trapezius and then the terminus, i.e., the lymph nodes below the scapula (see drawing on page 45).

---

4   The seventh cervical vertebra can be easily recognized because it corresponds to the bony elevation that appears when the neck is tilted forward.

Chapter 4

THE LYMPH NODES

GENERAL

FUNCTIONS

The lymph node can be compared to a station to which some lymphatic vessels (afferent) bring lymph and from which other vessels (efferent) take it away. The functions of the lymph node are basically threefold:

- filtering the incoming lymph, which is thus purified of the heaviest residues, and immunologically, of bacteria, viruses, fungi, and other harmful microorganisms present in the lymph;
- performing a valvular function, whereby the lymph node functions as a large valve preventing lymph reflux;
- performing a general immune function, with production of antibodies and cells designed to react specifically against infectious agents (immunocompetent cells).

The lymph nodes gather in lymph stations, consisting of two or more lymph nodes, established along the major lymphatic vessels.

Inside the organs, along the lymphatic capillaries, isolated cells (lymphocytes) function as a lymph node and are responsible for the production of antibodies. Alternatively, there are small cell groups comprising, in addition to lymphocytes, cells that form the inner lining of the capillaries and lymphatic vessels and that, in the event of infection, can transform into macrophages, i.e., cells that phagocytose infectious agents. In addition, these cell groups may include reticular cells that form a skeleton or support for the other cells of the same group.

If you consider the *grundsystem* (see pages 17–24), you will see the analogy between the *grundsystem* and the cell groups described above. Furthermore, the same typical organization of these cell groups and the *grundsystem* is found in the lymph node itself.

There are two types of lymph nodes:

- primary (almost exclusively for children);
- secondary (characteristic of adults; they are lymph nodes perfectly adapted to the body's various immune defenses).

FORM

The lymph node is roughly the shape of a dry bean. There is a convex part, called the *capsule*, which occupies almost two-thirds of the lymph node's surface, to which several lymphatic vessels reach and from which they carry the lymph to the lymph node; and also a slightly concave part, called the *hilum*, from which few lymphatic vessels or even a single one carries the lymph away. In larger lymph nodes, the outer surface, which is always smooth, may have some grooves, as if the lymph node were divided into smaller parts, called *lobules*.

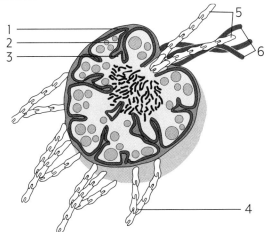

Lymph node in cross-section

1. Capsule
2. Peripheral lymphatic sinus
3. Capsular loop
4. Afferent (inflow) lymphatic vessels
5. Efferent (outflow) lymphatic vessels
6. Hilum artery and vein

DIMENSIONS AND NUMBER

Modern anatomical investigations have shown that the dimensions of lymph nodes can vary considerably, depending on the individual constitution, age, and physiological stage of the organism.

The diameter of a lymph node is only a few millimeters, but it can increase considerably in the case of infection or trauma, in which the lymph arrives with a toxic, bacterial, or viral load.

Lymph nodes are more voluminous in childhood and tend to shrink in size over the years.

It has been estimated that three thousand or more lymph nodes of different sizes can be found in the human body.

EXTERNAL APPEARANCE

Externally, the lymph node is white, especially in a young person. The inside, by contrast, is a darker, creamy white. In older people, the inner part has a yellowish color due to fat accumulation; in lung lymph nodes, especially in smokers and city dwellers, there are sometimes large black spots due to environmental pollution. The white outer zone is much more consistent than the creamy white inner zone, which is also more compact due to the number of connecting fibers, and which forms the capsule of the lymph node. A stalk-like vessel is attached to the concave part of the lymph node (hilum). Secondary lymph nodes can be recognized by the presence of two distinct zones: a darker peripheral one, populated almost exclusively by lymphocytes, and a central one, the so-called *light center* where plasma cells prevail.

APPEARANCE UNDER THE MICROSCOPE

THE CAPSULE

The outer surface of the lymph node is made up of overlapping layers of connecting fibers. In each layer the fibers run in different directions, which makes the capsule more resistant to the traction and compression that occur, for example, when the lymph node is enlarged or compressed near an organ.

The vessels that lead to the lymph node reach the capsule. After crossing it, they reach the lymphatic sinus, which is a space covered like the inner part of the vessels and which constitutes the first lymph purification chamber. In fact, the covering cells can be transformed into cells capable of absorbing toxic and infectious particles. The lymphatic sinus also performs the function of nourishing and purifying the lymph node.

Within the lymph node lie other lymph nodes that are spherical agglomerations consisting of hundreds or even thousands of lymphocytes, plasma cells, and dendritic cells.

LYMPHOCYTES

Lymphocytes are cells grown in the thymus, which is a kind of large lymph gland located beneath the thyroid. Thanks to their membrane, lymphocytes carry antibodies specific to a type of bacteria, virus, or other pathogen (whether infectious or even toxic) with which the organism has come into contact. When a pathogen reaches the lymph node, lymphocytes specialized to fight it surround and attack it.

PLASMA CELLS

Plasma cells are large cells that, unlike lymphocytes, do not attack the pathogen directly, but produce specific antibodies to destroy it.

DENDRITIC CELLS

Dendritic cells (from the Greek word *dendron*, meaning "branch," because of their branched appearance) are special reticular cells that form a support structure for lymphocytes and plasma cells.

Thanks to their shape, dendritic cells create microscopic channels[5] into which lymph, originating in the lymphatic sinus, enters, allowing it to come into contact with the cells of the immune system so as to provide specific defenses.

THE MEDULLARY REGION

From the outermost part of the lymph node, the lymph reaches the medullary region, which constitutes approximately one-third of the lymph node volume.

The vessels originating from the hilum of the lymph node are located in this region. As the lymph is directed there, first the walls of the capillaries and then those of the lymphatic vessels become individualized, close to the venous and arterial vessels. Fewer lymphatic vessels leave the hilum than reach the capsule.

---

5 To get an idea of size, think of a channel formed by dendritic cells that is estimated to have an average diameter of just 200 angstroms (1 Å = 0.000001 mm).

From the collarbone or clavicle

Subclavian (just below the clavicle, at the lateral margin of the small pectoralis muscle). It collects lymph from the axillary lymph nodes. In some cases, the subclavian duct can be isolated.

Supraclavicular. It is located in the lesser supraclavicular fossa, between the medial and lateral insertion tendons of the sterno-cleidomastoid muscle, where the lymph from the subclavian lymph nodes, the subclavian lymphatic duct, and the jugular lymphatic duct of the head converge, near the mouth of the thoracic duct and the bronchomediastinal duct into the subclavian vein.

Axillary. It is a complex lymphatic station, including several lymphonodal stations.

Station below the shoulder blade that collects lymph from the large superficial muscles of the back—the latissimus dorsi and trapezius in particular—the lower cervical region and much of the breast.

Brachial station. This is where the lymph from the arm is collected. It is located around the subclavian vein at its entry into the axillary hollow.

Central axillary station. It collects lymph from the brachial lymph nodes and from below the scapula and originates lymphatic collectors directed towards the station below the scapula.

Interpectoral or Rotter's lymph nodes. This is a network of lymph nodes located inside the large pectoralis muscle, where lymph from the pectoralis muscle and the upper part of the breast is collected.

Internal or parasternal mammary station. It is composed of a chain of 6 to 10 lymph nodes located parallel to the edge of the sternum, at a distance of 1 to 2 cm, along the thoracic muscular insertions of the large pectoral muscle and above the costal arch, in the lower part of the sternum. The right station collects lymph from the right medial part of the breast, the medial part of the large pectoralis, and the sternal region and sends lymphatic vessels to the left station, which is tributary to the thoracic duct. However, it can also form an autonomous trunk superiorly, which enters directly into the subclavian duct on the right and the thoracic duct on the left; the lower lymph nodes of the chain collect lymphatic vessels from the anterior part of the diaphragm and, on the right, from the liver.

Drainage Areas	Related Disorders
Neck and head homolaterally, arm and breast homolaterally	Headache, neck stiffness, cervical osteoarthritis; general head and neck disorders; arm, back, and breast disorders
Arm, breast, and dorsal region	Shoulder pain, plus topathy, breast tension, breast cyst, shoulder arthrosis, arm, and elbow pain (epicondylitis).
Large and small pectoral, upper part of breast	Some straining of the pectoral muscles may cause swelling of these lymph nodes, which may suggest the presence of breast lymph nodes.
Medial part of the large pectoralis and breast muscle, sternal region, and medial part of the intercostal spaces; anterior part of the diaphragm; left anterior part of the liver	Sprains and strains of the pectoralis muscle can cause a bulging of these lymph nodes, which can look like medial breast nodes. Also the suffering of medial breast lymph nodes can cause lymph node enlargement in this region.

Inguinal (located along the inguinal ligament); it can be divided into four main sectors:

- upper medial sector (collects lymph from the abdominal wall and external genitalia);
- upper lateral sector (collects lymph from the lateral two-thirds of the abdominal wall and buttocks);
- lower medial sector (collects lymph from the superficial circulation of the leg);
- lower lateral sector (collects lymph that runs parallel to the deep venous vessels)

Submaxillary. It is situated below the mandible, occupies the posterior three-quarters of the retromandibular space; it collects lymph from the station below the chin and sends it to the inferior auricular or angulus station.

Under the chin. It lies in front of the submaxillary lymph nodes; from here the lymph reaches the lymph nodes of the submaxillary station.

Anterior auricular or parotid. It is located in front of the auricle of the ear, in the parotid region. The lymph goes to the inferior auricular or angulus station, also called *profundus* in lymphatic drainage terminology.

Posterior auricular or mastoid. Located behind the pinna, in the mastoid region.

Drainage Areas	Related Disorders
Leg, bladder, genital organs, pelvis	Pain in the pubis, hip, lumbosacral region, leg problems, venous insufficiency of the leg
Mandible, mandibular sinus (together with the anterior auricular or parotid station), mouth, posterior part of tongue, teeth and gums of the mandible, except incisors; fangs and premolars of the upper jaw, part of the upper lip, narib, lacrimal ganglia, medial part of the orbital region and eye	Discomfort in the mouth, teeth, gums, nose, sinuses, eye (with poor or excessive lacrimation), lingual and submaxillary salivary glands (dryness or excessive saliva production).
Anterior quarter of the mandible, upper and lower incisor teeth, anterior half of the tongue, lower lip, and part of upper lip	Discomfort of the lips and incisor teeth, aphthae (small ovoid erosions of the mucous membrane of the mouth) located in the region of the incisors
Temporomandibular joint (TMJ), front of the head, lateral part of the eye, parotid, upper molars, ear	Trigeminal neuralgia, migraine, temporofrontal headache, nodular headache, parotitis (mumps), ear complaints, tinnitus (ringing and whistling), otitis, tooth infections or problems, dislocation of the jaw, dental occlusion problems, bruxism
Central part of the head, temporal and parietal regions, ear, mastoid, eighth tooth (wisdom tooth), retromolar space	Infections or problems with wisdom teeth, otitis, migraine, mastoid infections

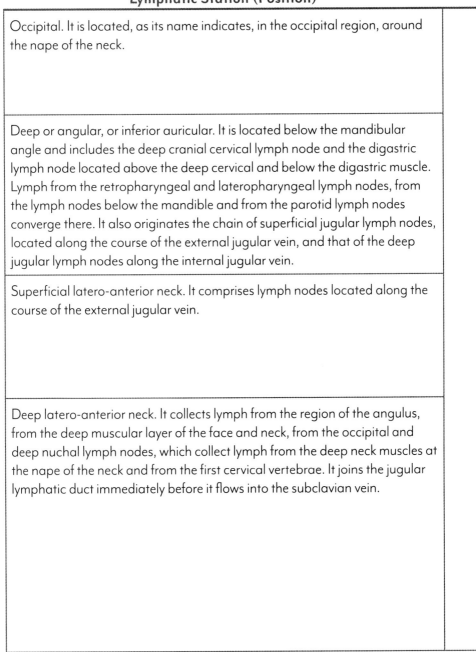

Occipital. It is located, as its name indicates, in the occipital region, around the nape of the neck.

Deep or angular, or inferior auricular. It is located below the mandibular angle and includes the deep cranial cervical lymph node and the digastric lymph node located above the deep cervical and below the digastric muscle. Lymph from the retropharyngeal and lateropharyngeal lymph nodes, from the lymph nodes below the mandible and from the parotid lymph nodes converge there. It also originates the chain of superficial jugular lymph nodes, located along the course of the external jugular vein, and that of the deep jugular lymph nodes along the internal jugular vein.

Superficial latero-anterior neck. It comprises lymph nodes located along the course of the external jugular vein.

Deep latero-anterior neck. It collects lymph from the region of the angulus, from the deep muscular layer of the face and neck, from the occipital and deep nuchal lymph nodes, which collect lymph from the deep neck muscles at the nape of the neck and from the first cervical vertebrae. It joins the jugular lymphatic duct immediately before it flows into the subclavian vein.

Drainage Areas	Related Disorders
Occipital region, nape of neck, first cervical vertebra	Occipital headache, nuchal headache, heaviness in the back of the neck, loss of balance, lipotimia (fainting) caused by sudden head movements
Pharynx, throat, retromolar space, lymph from auricular and posterior lymph nodes, submaxillary lymph nodes	Discomfort in the throat, pharynx, palatine, tubal and pharyngeal tonsils
Neck muscles, lymph from the inferior auricular or angular station. They converge in the key lymph nodes or form a single duct, the jugular duct, which enters directly into the subclavian vein.	Torticollis and discomfort of the masticatory and paramasticatory musculature; reduced neck mobility
Anterolateral deep muscular layer of the neck: pharynx, larynx, esophagus. It comprises the lymph nodes of the internal jugular chain, situated along the internal jugular vein. The transverse jugular chain, located parallel to the upper edge of the clavicle. the spinal nerve chain, situated along the course of the spinal nerve itself, running approximately perpendicular to the clavicle, exiting from the angle of the clavicle.	Inflammatory discomfort in the neck organs (pharynx, larynx, esophagus), which may even cause stiffness in the neck muscles, from the deep muscles

Superficial anterior neck: includes the subcutaneous lymph nodes located in the anterior neck; the lymph flows into the jugular duct.

Anterior deep anterior neck. It comprises supra- and infra-hyoid lymph nodes, whose lymph flows respectively into the lateral lymphatic chains of the neck in the lymph nodes situated in the sternum—pre- and paratracheal lymph nodes—from which the lymph reaches the pre-mediastinal lymph nodes situated in the thorax, below the sternum, tributaries of the broncho-mediastinal trunk, which then flows into the subclavian lymph nodes.

Lymphatic system of the breast. The lymphatic network is made up of small, very fine vessels located near the breast areola and in the interglandular connective tissue.

Ulnar or elbow

Drainage Areas	Related Disorders
Subcutis and superficial muscles of the front of the neck	Allergic skin manifestations of the anterior neck. Other skin complaints arising from adjacent organs, particularly the larynx and thyroid, are also frequent.
Anterior deep muscles of the neck, larynx, trachea, thyroid and parathyroid, esophagus	Inflammations of the larynx (laryngitis), trachea (tracheitis), esophagus (esophagitis, often present in case of hiatus hernia, due to acid regurgitations from the stomach), thyroid (thyroiditis, often present in proximity to inflammations of the larynx and trachea).
The main outflow route is to the lymph nodes under the scapula and the axilla. The lymphatic vessels from the upper part of the breast are partly directed to the interpectoral lymph nodes and from there to the subclavian lymph nodes. The medial lymphatic vessels are partly directed to the parasternal or internal mammary lymph nodes. The course of the lymphatic vessels of the breast suggests the importance of the condition of the back and the pectoralis muscle.	Back problems, usually associated with reduced respiratory function and pectoral muscle fatigue, easily lead to lymphatic stasis of the breast, facilitating the formation of nodules and various types of pathology, including glandular tissue.
Elbow, forearm, wrist, hand	Elbow pain, inflammation of the epicondyle and epicondylitis, Dupuytre's morbus, carpal tunnel syndrome, paresthesias of the hands.

Lymphatic Station (Position)

Popliteal or knee. The lymph nodes are distributed in three layers: the deep lymph nodes collect lymph from the knee itself. The middle lymph nodes collect lymph from the deep circulation of the leg, ankle, and foot. The superficial lymph nodes are satellites of the superficial venous system and collect lymph from the subcutis of the knee and the underlying parts.	
Perineal	
Paravertebral. The lymph nodes located laterally to each vertebra	
Pecquet's cistern. The intestinal duct, which collects lymph from the digestive and intestinal organs, and the iliac ducts, which collect lymph from the legs and pelvic organs, flow into it.	
Thoracic duct. Collects lymph from Pecquet's cistern and the chest wall; when the right great lymphatic vein is present, it collects lymph only from the left side of the chest wall.	
Right large lymphatic vein (often absent)	
Jugular duct	
Broncho-diastinal duct	
Subclavian duct	

Drainage Areas	Related Disorders
Knee, leg, ankle, and foot	Knee pain, meniscus pain, osteoarthritis of the knee, ankle dislocations, foot pain, and deformities
Genitalia, rectum, perineal muscles	Anerosias, dysmenorrhoea, rectocolitis, haemorrhoids, epididymitis, etc.
Bone, periosteal, cartilaginous, muscular and nervous territories of each vertebra	Vertebral pain and deformities, herniated discs, osteoporosis, pleurisy
Legs, pelvis, abdominal organs, abdominal wall below the umbilicus (navel)	Problems in the legs, pelvis, abdominal organs, lumbosacral pains
Legs, abdominal organs, chest wall	As in Pecquet's cistern, adding discomfort due to pain, chest wall trauma, dorsal scoliosis, etc.
Lymph from the right side of the chest wall	Chest pains and deformities, particularly on the right side of the chest
Lymph from one-half of the head	Lymph from one-half of the head
Lymph from the right or left half of the organs of the thorax and mediastinum	Discomfort in the heart, lungs, pleura, lungs, and pleura
Lymph from the right or left arm	Discomfort in the arms

HOW TO KEEP THE LYMPHATIC SYSTEM IN SHAPE

Chapter 5

LYMPHATIC DRAINAGE

GENERAL

Lymphatic drainage consists of facilitating the circulation of lymph through the lymphatic vessels and lymph nodes. This is achieved by exerting light pressure along the lymphatic pathways and on the intervening lymphonodal stations.

As noted above, the body's lymph flows in the subclavian veins, near the angle they form with the external jugular vein, in a small area. Emil Vodder, a Dane who created a description of modern lymphatic drainage, called this area the *terminus*, which comprises two distinct areas: the left and the right. The left terminus is the most important, as this is where the lymph from the abdominal organs, legs, abdominal wall, and thoracic wall arrives.

Vodder established that every drainage treatment had to start by emptying the terminus—to allow the body's lymph to flow freely toward this point—and he also determined that the main lympho-nodal stations of the head, as a lymphatic stasis in the head, can easily block the drainage. This last possibility explains why cigarette smoke, especially in women, can facilitate the formation of cellu-litis in the legs and pelvis: in fact, the lymphatic stasis created in the terminus by chronic inflammation of the throat slows down the lymphatic flow from the legs.

To conclude: the lymph drainage practitioner has to facilitate the circulation of lymph in the head and the terminus; only then can he or she move on to the specific treatment of, for example, the legs or arms, abdomen, thorax, face, cranial vault, back, and other body parts.

CONTRAINDICATIONS

Since most diseases are associated with lymphatic stasis, many ailments can benefit from lymphatic drainage.

In the case of acute illness, accompanied by fever and symptoms of infection, the emptying of the lymph nodes could facilitate dangerous bacterial and viral loads moving into general circulation.

Lymph drainage is also not recommended when there is a suspicion or certainty of a neoplasm (cancer), as the emptying of the lymph nodes would encourage the spread of diseased cells throughout the body.

EFFECTS OF DRAINAGE

REDUCTION OF EDEMA, SWELLING, AND CELLULITE

Edema, swelling, and cellulitis occur wherever there is lymphatic stasis, as a result of the following disorders:

- kidney and liver diseases;
- venous insufficiency (especially in the legs);
- premenstrual period;
- pregnancy;
- termination of lactation (swelling of the breast can even be painful and cause mastitis);

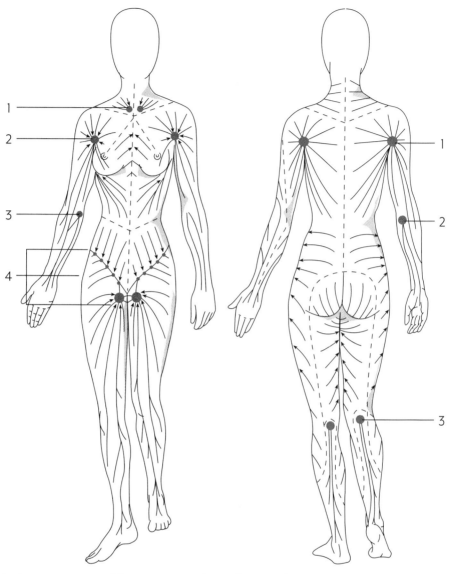

In this representation of the anterior part of the body, there is a diagram summarizing the distribution of the lymphatic vessels and circulation. The points indicate the main lymphonodal stations.

1. Key lymph nodes
2. Axillary lymph nodes
3. Lymph nodes of the elbow
4. Inguinal lymph nodes

Diagram showing the main lymphonodal stations, the distribution of vessels, and lymphatic circulation in the posterior part of the body.

1. Axillary lymph nodes
2. Elbow lymph nodes
3. Knee lymph nodes

- seasonal change between spring and summer (usually in conjunction with venous insufficiency);
- spending a long time in an upright position;
- a consequence of trauma.

The reduction of swelling also corresponds to a purification of the related tissue, caused by the removal of waste products with the lymph.

IMMUNE STIMULATION AND RAPID HEALING

These effects appear together following the removal of waste and the stimulation of the immune system of the lymph nodes.

Lymphatic drainage stimulates wound healing and proper healing, accelerating the healing process and reducing the risk of keloid formation (excessive scar tissue).

Drainage is very useful in the following cases:

- postoperative period;
- to prevent bedsores in the elderly or those who are bedridden for long periods;
- burns;
- trauma;
- varicose ulcers.

STIMULATION OF MICROCIRCULATION

This is a very beneficial effect of lymphatic drainage, particularly in cases of the following:

- peripheral circulation disorders (characterized by hands or feet that are always cold);
- chilblains;
- Raynaud's syndrome;
- Buerger's disease (smoker's disease).

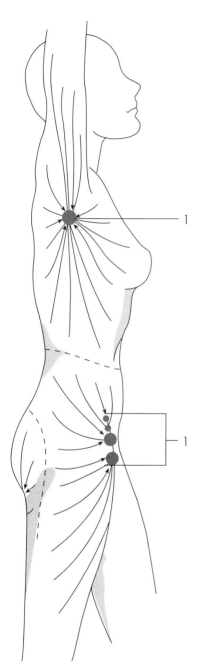

Diagram of the lymph nodes, vessel distribution, and lymphatic circulation in the lateral part of the body. Note the clear separation between the areas that send lymph to the axillary lymph nodes and those that send it to the inguinal lymph nodes.

1. Axillary lymph nodes
2. Inguinal lymph nodes

REJUVENATION

The rejuvenating function of lymph drainage is particularly noticeable in a new appearance of the skin, which looks younger thanks to the removal of waste products through the lymphatic system and the consequent reduction of the horny layer of the epidermis (which absorbs light, giving the skin a darker and dirtier appearance). In addition, the improvement of the subcutaneous microcirculation, by reducing the evidence of wrinkles, makes the skin more luminous.

TONICITY

After drainage, thanks to the removal of waste and improved microcirculation, fatigue is often relieved and sleep becomes deep and more restorative. Lymph drainage thus eliminates one of the most unpleasant effects of busy city life: the feeling of constant tiredness, which makes daily activities more tiring than usual.

RELAXATION

If the drainage is well done, the feeling of well-being produced in the patient is one of pleasant relaxation, lightness, and freshness. Drainage therefore relaxes, combats anxiety, and promotes sleep.

MAIN CLINICAL INDICATIONS FOR LYMPHATIC DRAINAGE

ONCOLOGY

In oncology, or the field of cancer, lymphatic drainage finds a good application in mastectomized women who often suffer from painful lymphedema of the inner arm that which may be caused by the ablation of the axillary lymph nodes. In this case, the normal flow of lymph from the arm along the subclavian lymphatic duct to the terminus is blocked.

To solve this problem, massage can be used to stimulate the lymphatic vessels in the back and increase the flow to the contralateral (opposite side) axilla, so that lymph from the damaged arm goes to the contralateral subclavian duct.

It has been observed, in fact, that prolonged gentle pushing on the lymphatic vessels can even reverse the direction of flow through the channels. Thus, the lymphatic vessels in the dorsal region of one side of the body, whose flow normally goes to the axilla, reverse their direction of flow to the contralateral axilla, as a result of the prolonged lymphatic drainage.

ESTHETIC MEDICINE

One of the best-known applications of lymph drainage is a treatment to tone the skin, especially the complexion, as it unblocks lymphatic stasis and promotes blood microcirculation and rapid tissue renewal. Those processes help prevent the formation of bags and wrinkles on the face, reduce the horny layer of the epidermis, and give the face a much smoother and more luminous appearance.

ACNE

Acne is a widespread phenomenon in adolescence, affecting mainly the skin of the face (in particular the forehead, chin, and cheeks) as well as the shoulders and chest (area between the breasts). Acne can also occur in other areas on the upper part of the body.

This happens, according to traditional Chinese medicine, because the "yin" in the liver is weak and fails to stop the "yang," which, being hot, rises and accumulates in the face.[6]

According to Western medical criteria, the yin of the liver corresponds approximately to the metabolic processes of fat transformation and the formation of bile, which, on the one hand, is a means of removing waste products (mainly from fat and blood metabolism) and, on the other hand, helps to emulsify fats resulting from digestion. When the yin is poured into the duodenum, it contributes significantly to its assimilation. Imperfect digestion and defective fat metabolism lead to a disturbance of the intestinal flora, with the consequent occurrence of abnormal fermentation and putrefaction processes in the intestine, resulting in a general rise in body temperature, especially in the upper parts of the body. The heat of the ascending liver would be the yang. The reason for the liver to let the yang escape is its increased "tiredness" during adolescence, due to the increased hormone production that the metabolism has to cope with.

The first cure for acne is a diet free of fats, fried foods, sausages, sweets, and alcoholic beverages. It is better to abstain from snacks, martinis, pizzas, and sweet drinks and to replace milk with yogurt.

---

6   See page 185 for an explanation of the concepts of yin and yang.

Once the regime has been corrected, lymphatic drainage offers an important aid, as it facilitates the removal of the fatty "plugs" that close the sebaceous lymph nodes of the face and cause the characteristic lesions of acne. This is especially true in the case of comedones, which can appear in the form of either blackheads (due to phenomena of oxidation of the fat or deposition of dust particles) or whiteheads (when the sebaceous lymph node closed by the fatty plug is close to infectious processes, accompanied by the production of pus). If the comedones spread to the subcutaneous tissue, they can cause, in order of severity, papules, pustules, and phlegmons; their healing can lead to the formation of unsightly scars.

In conclusion, lymphatic drainage, after following a balanced diet and aesthetic cleansing of the face, can reduce acne formations until they disappear. During successive treatments, they disappear first from the upper parts of the face (forehead), then from the intermediate parts (cheeks), and finally from the lower parts (chin and submaxillary region), while the lymph loaded with residues goes toward the terminus.

COSMETIC SURGERY

Lymphatic drainage is present in all cosmetic surgery (in particular *facelifts*) and plastic surgery of the face, reducing or preventing scar formation and accelerating tissue healing times. For example, lymphatic drainage is used after correction of the ears to promote healing, as it helps the auricular lymph nodes to expel waste products toward the terminus.

Lymphatic drainage, in addition, also favors the healing of skin areas that have undergone surgery, thereby avoiding the risk of keloids (large, raised scars).

DENTISTRY AND OTORHINOLARYNGOLOGY

In dentistry, lymphatic drainage of the gums is used to support ortho-dontics (i.e., the corrective shifting of teeth), especially in children, and sometimes also in adults.

In otorhinolaryngology, lymphatic drainage facilitates the reduction of lymphatic stasis and, consequently, of the tenacious catarrh present in chronic inflammations of the nose, paranasal sinuses, and throat, which favors their healing.

For this purpose, in addition to lymphatic drainage, inhalations should be carried out. The inhaler device emits hot steam with a few drops of emulsifying essential oil that has been previously poured into a glass of water; this helps to keep the stubborn cold at bay and disinfects the mucous membranes. The most commonly used essential oil is eucalyptus. Inhalation should not be confused with aerosol spraying, which emits cold medicinal particles. Although it is very useful in the acute (hot) phase, with heavy colds, it is not recommended in the treatment of chronic cold conditions, in which it causes excessive dryness of the mucous membranes and thus impedes healing.

There is also a home version of the commercial inhaler devices, which consists of positioning one's head carefully over a pot of boiling water containing a few drops of eucalyptus oil and covering the head with a towel. This is not suitable for children, as the steam tends to irritate the skin and eyes.

ORTHOPEDICS

In orthopedics, lymphatic drainage is very useful in the reeducation of motor skills after joint immobilization, as it considerably reduces functional recovery times and improves results.

Lymph drainage also has an effective application in all chronic processes affecting bones and joints—such as arthrosis, for example—

as it helps to prevent the worsening of pathological phenomena and sometimes even leads to an improvement. In addition, it is useful in the treatment of contusions, epicondylitis, and epitrochleitis, as well as in sprains and, in general, in tendon and ligament injuries.

SPORTS MEDICINE

In sports medicine, apart from the advantages mentioned above, good lymph drainage allows for a faster recovery of the athlete's musculature after agonistic fatigue. It becomes indispensable, combined with muscle massage, in the prevention of muscle strains, which tend to occur more easily in athletes suffering from lymphatic stasis in the limbs or other parts of the body caused by previous problems.

ANGIOLOGY

The best-known indication for lymphatic drainage, apart from the treatment of the face, is the treatment of lymphatic and venous stasis in the legs—in particular, cellulite on the thighs and pelvis, caused by dentistry, poor diet, irregular menstruation, smoking, and the use of drugs (see pages 161–173).

It should be remembered that minimal or even lack of cellulite is of great aesthetic importance, but it also indicates the presence of a more or less pronounced venous insufficiency that lymphatic drainage can prevent and cure, thus avoiding a worsening after its manifestation.

DRAINAGE TECHNIQUE

THE MOVEMENTS

On the face, light pressure can be applied with the fingertips, while on the trunk and limbs, the fingers and palms of the hands should be used.

The pressure exerted varies from a few grams (over the most delicate areas of the face) to a maximum of 50 grams (on the trunk and limbs).

Normally, the drainage thrust is applied in the physiological direction of lymph drainage (see pages 69–71), describing semi-circles. In the beginning, the pressure exerted should always be very light. As the person doing the treatment moves forward, she or he must increase the pressure until it reaches its maximum in the middle part (the apex of the arc) and decrease it until it disappears at the end of the semicircle. There, the draining part (the fingers and hands) is lifted, quickly marking a second semicircle, at the end of which it is placed back on top of the patient and the treating person (the therapist) starts again.

Basically, using the fingers or the hand, the therapist marks a circle; in one-half the therapist does the actual pushing, while the other half is used to maintain the rhythm and harmony of the drainage.

Actually, it would be fairer to speak of pressing in spirals rather than circles, in order to make the most of the arrangement of the lymphatic valves, which are arranged along the lymphatic vessels in a slightly spiral shape. For this reason, the main direction of the thrust in each semicircle must be slightly different from the previous one, but always around the main axis. Sometimes they may overlap with each other or be linked one after the other.

NUMBER OF MOVEMENTS

At each point, between one and five movements are usually made, depending on the lymphatic stasis of the area exposed to drainage. Naturally, in those areas where lymph tends to accumulate, it will be necessary for the therapist to press with more emphasis. Each pressure should be made in a slightly different direction from the previous one, following a spiral path.

RHYTHM OF MOVEMENTS

Each movement should be performed after a two- to three-second pause, to promote the physiological rhythm of contraction of the muscle cells arranged along the vessel walls.

VARIETY OF PRESSURE TECHNIQUES

Sometimes, as in some operations on the head, face, and fingers of the hand, in contrast to the previous cases, a light-oriented digital pressure is used, while the therapist keeps the fingers still.

In other cases, as in the treatment of the supraciliary region, a small pinch is performed.

In the treatment of the upper orbital region (under the eyebrows), a small upward traction is performed, keeping the fingers on the same skin area, which causes a pulling movement. Another effective technique is to rub the forehead superficially. As this area is almost completely devoid of subcutaneous tissue, the rubbing is enough to stimulate the lymphatic vessels.

The rubbing is also applied to the abdomen, following the course of the colon, in the shape of an open horseshoe pointing downward, to stimulate intestinal transit and overcome constipation.

Finally, during the treatment of the face, the heat produced by the therapist's open hands is used to relieve possible spasms of the lymphatic vessels of the face and forehead.

DEVELOPMENT OF PERCEPTIONS

The therapist's skill depends, in addition to his or her anatomical and physiological knowledge of the lymphatic system and the movements that help the lymph to circulate, on a particular intuitive sensitivity. In the most attentive therapists, this sensitivity is the product of long experience that allows them to adapt the pressure and rhythm of the treatment to the characteristics of each patient.

THE PHASES OF EACH TREATMENT

Every treatment, even on a limited area of the body, should consists of the following steps:

- emptying of the lymph nodes of the head, neck, and terminus;
- treatment of the body part in question;
- drainage of the most important lymph nodes between the treated area and the terminus;
- emptying of the terminus.

For example, if drainage of the right elbow is desired, the head and neck will be treated first and then the right terminus. Then the lymph nodes of the elbow and axilla are drained and, finally, the right terminus is drained again.

MECHANICAL AND ELECTRICAL MEANS FOR LYMPHATIC DRAINAGE

The following chapter will describe in detail the techniques of manual lymphatic drainage, which is probably the most effective way of stimulating the movement of lymph. For the time being, we will briefly discuss other means used in lymph drainage, both mechanical and electrical. Obviously, it is impossible to ask of an instrument the precision achieved by manual drainage carried out by a good therapist.

MECHANICAL INSTRUMENTS

These are cuffs that, when connected to a compressor, provide a rhythmic and coordinated pressure of the lymph, especially in the legs.

However, prior to the application of this system, it is necessary to manually decongest the terminus and regional lymph nodes. In addition, this procedure requires constant attention from the therapist to ensure that the thrust is proportionate to the individual complexion and follows the desired direction.

INSTRUMENTS FOR ELECTROSTIMULATION

These means of electrical stimulation are used for muscle activation in motor reeducation and sports training. If used correctly, they provide a good aid to manual drainage, as the muscle contraction provoked by these means exerts a physiological push on the lymphatic vessels.

By means of these instruments the therapist can monitor all the reactions of the patient, manually intervening in the emptying of the terminus and the lymph nodes of the body part being treated.

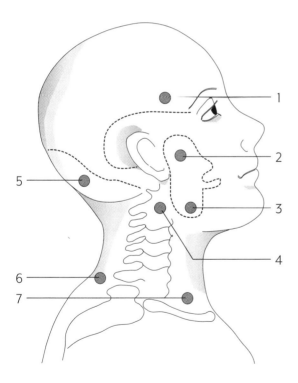

The diagram shows the points to act on at the beginning of drainage, prior to any treatment.

1. Temporal lymph nodes

2. Anterior parotid or auricular lymph nodes

3. Anteroinferior auricular lymph nodes

4. Inferior auricular lymph nodes

5. Occipital lymph nodes

6. Upper trapezius lymph nodes

7. Key lymph nodes and lymphatic duct outflow into the subclavian vein

Chapter 6

HOW TO PERFORM MANUAL LYMPHATIC DRAINAGE

This chapter describes in detail how a complete lymph drainage session is carried out on all parts of the body.

The previous chapter has already described the necessary movements required to exert the appropriate pressure, as well as the ideal duration and the rhythm of the pressure.

START

As already mentioned, any lymphatic drainage session must be preceded by a preliminary phase in which the lymphonodal chains of the head, neck, and, of course, the terminus are treated.

1. It starts with an emptying of the auricular lymph nodes.

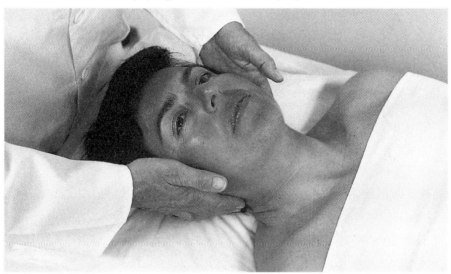

2. Lymph is then pushed from the auricular lymph nodes to the laterocervical lymph nodes and from there to the terminus.

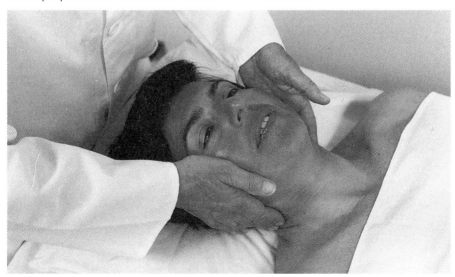

3. The termus is emptied.

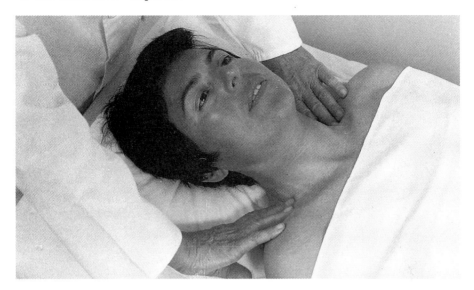

4. The occipital lymph nodes are emptied.

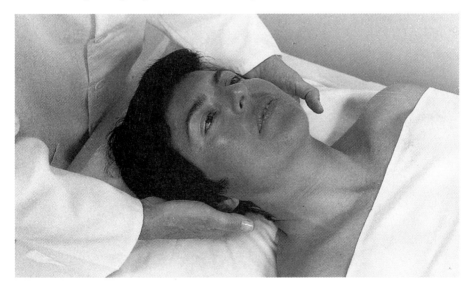

5. The cervical lymph nodes are emptied.

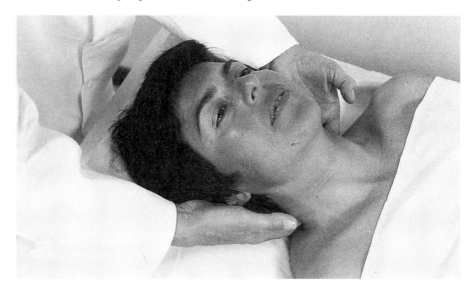

6. The lymph nodes of the trapezium are emptied.

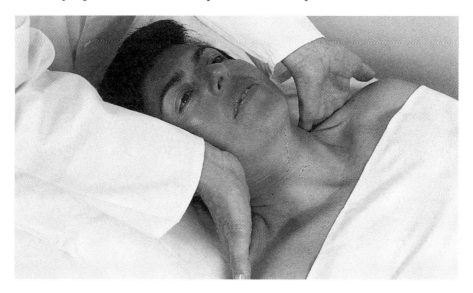

7. The submaxillary lymph nodes are emptied.

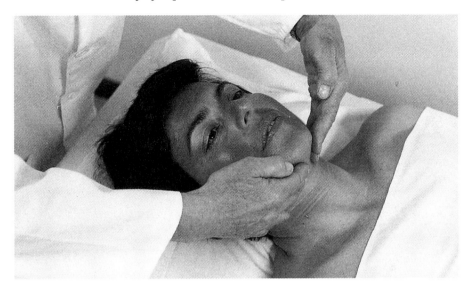

8. Finally, the temporal lymph nodes are emptied.

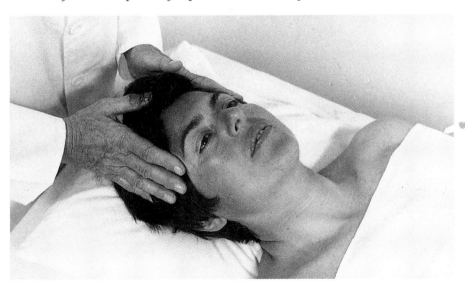

9. The second treatment of the auricular lymph nodes is then carried out.

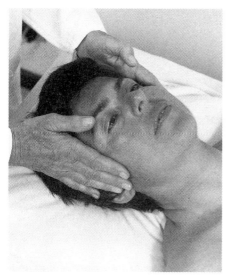 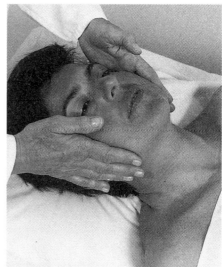

10. Start by emptying the profundus.

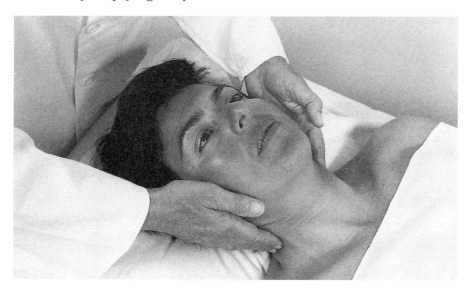

11. And the terminus is emptied again.

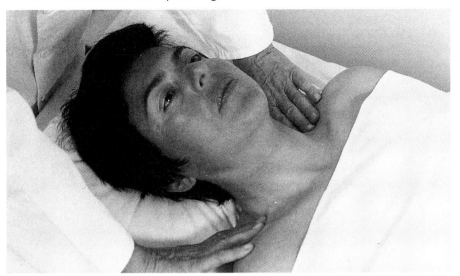

FIRST TREATMENT OF THE FACE (ANTEROLATERAL SIDE)

1. Start at the chin and lower lip. The pushing movement is used to allow the lymph to flow toward the submaxillary lymph nodes.

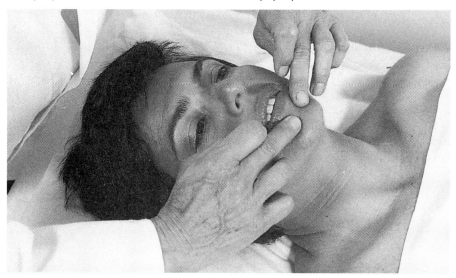

2. The submaxillary lymph node is emptied.

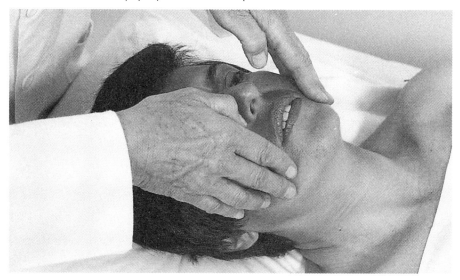

3. Then the nodes between the nose and the lips are emptied.

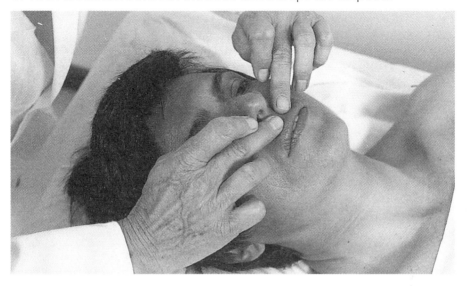

4. The parotid lymph nodes are emptied.

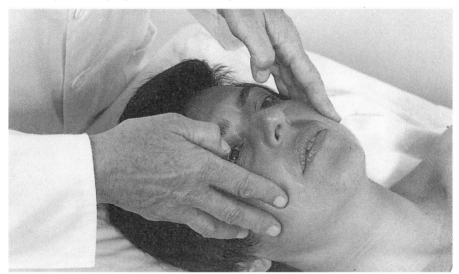

5. When treating the nose, the fingers describe five semicircles in the following areas.

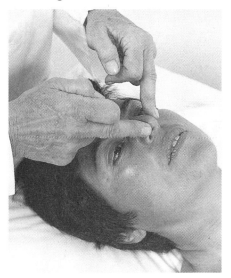
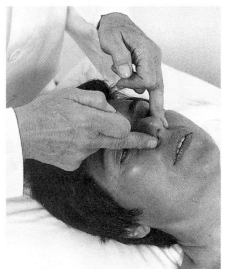
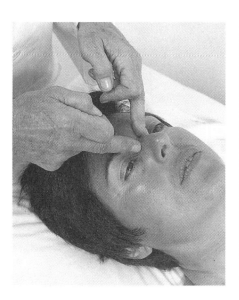
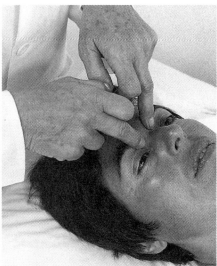

6. The fingers are held still above the cheeks and oriented as if to press gently vertically and outward. At the same time, the palm of the hand, barely separated, emits a pleasant warmth on the upper part of the face and forehead, avoiding the spasms that could affect the muscles of the vessels and impede normal circulation.

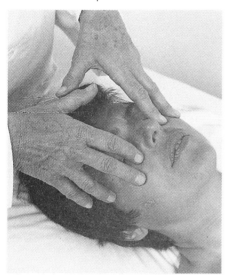 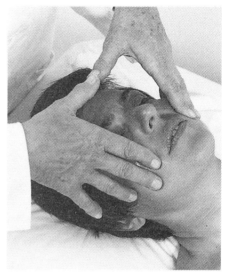

7. Emptying of the submaxillary lymph nodes, to which the lymph has been directed by the previous movements.

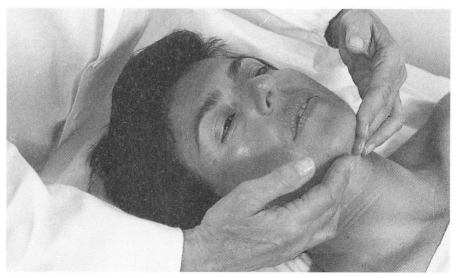

8. Treatment of the eyebrows, using a light pinch for approximately two seconds, from the inside to the outside.

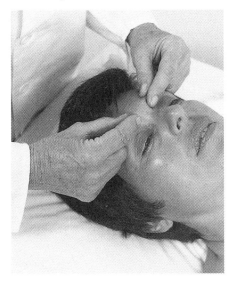 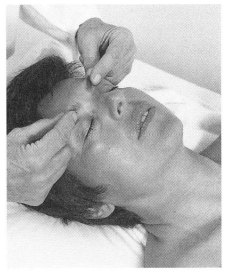

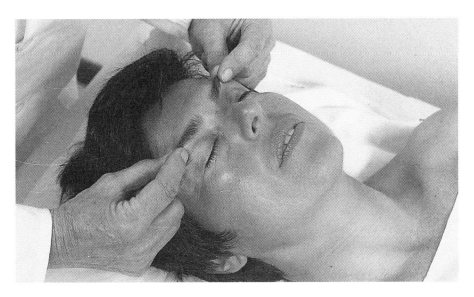

9. Treatment of the upper part of the orbit is also very useful for subocular "bags." A slight upward traction is made with the index finger, starting from the upper inner corner of the orbit. The other fingers, except the thumb, are placed on the inferior margin, exerting very light pressure. A few seconds later, they must be placed one after the other, from the third to the fifth finger.

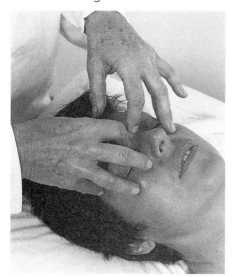 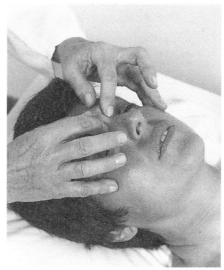

10. At the same time, the hands open upward like the corolla of a flower, until they rest on the temples with the margin of the fifth finger at the level of the metacarpus, exerting a pressure that allows the emptying of the temporal lymph nodes.

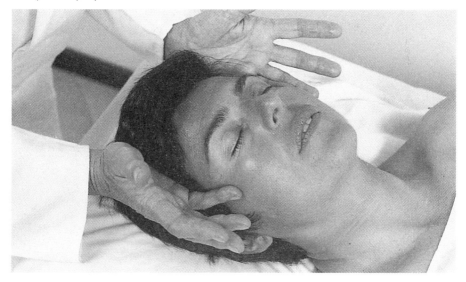

11. Treatment of the forehead and the region adjacent to the scalp is carried out with a direct touch behind .

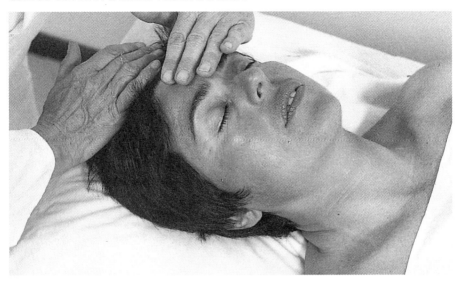

12. Treatment of the parietal region is then initiated.

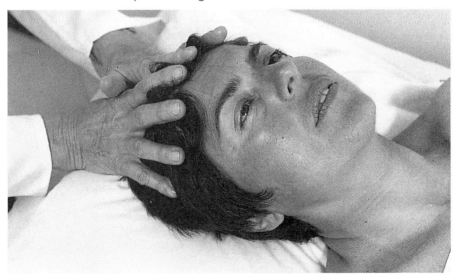

13. Treatment of the temporal and superior auricular lymph nodes is continued.

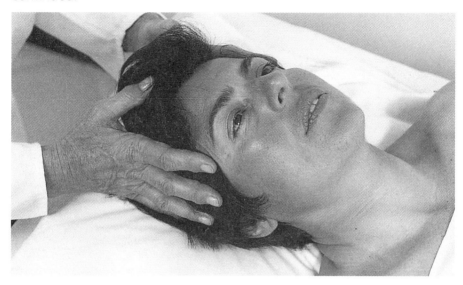

14. Treatment of the parotid lymph nodes is continued.

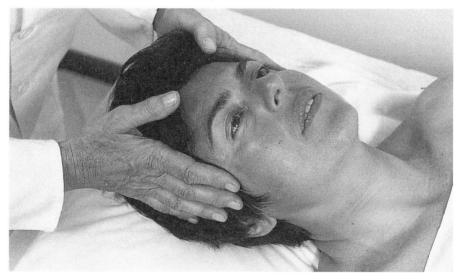

15. The auricular lymph nodes are emptied.

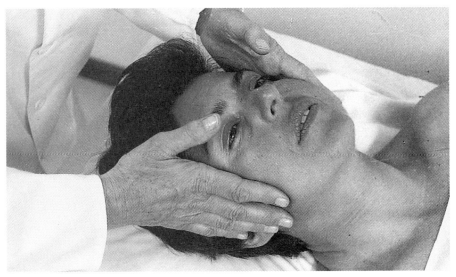

16. The profundus (lower auricular lymph nodes) is emptied.

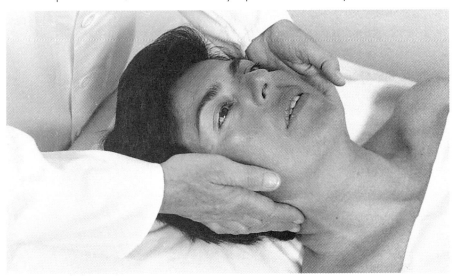

17. And finally, the terminus is emptied. This operation completes the treatment of the anterolateral part of the face.

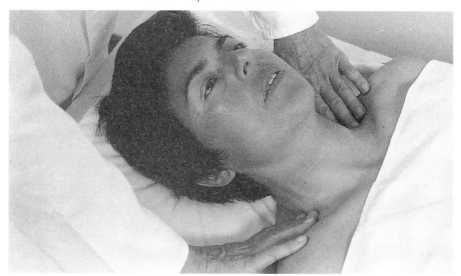

SECOND TREATMENT OF THE FACE (FRONTAL AND OCCIPITAL PARTS)

1. To begin, proceed from the top downward, with the hands open. The tips of the index fingers, which are almost together at the beginning, move away from each other as you descend.

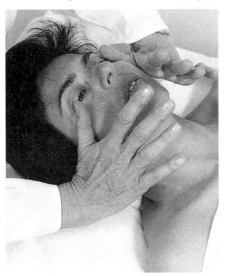 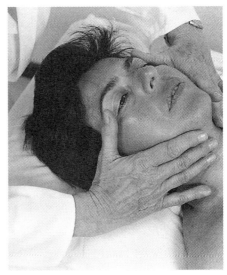

2. Then proceed from the sides, from the top downward and from the inside outward. The extremities of the thumbs are together above the forehead and then spread apart as they descend.

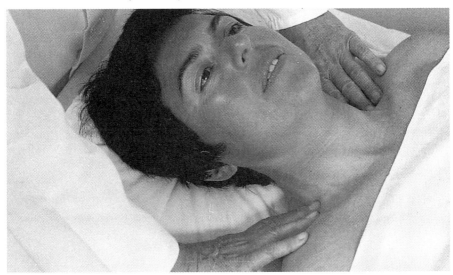

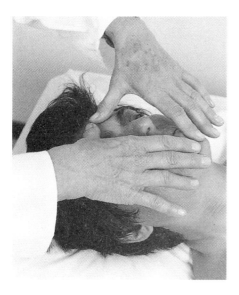
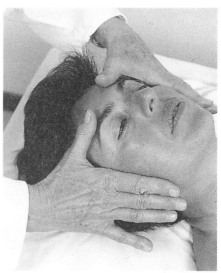

3. The occipital region is treated from top to bottom.

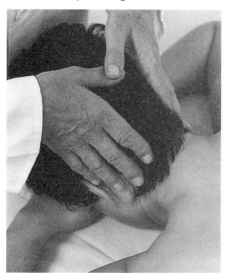
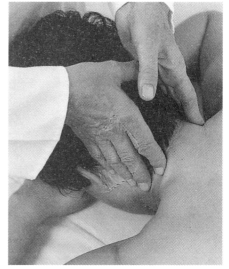

4. The second treatment of the face and occipital region is completed with the emptying of the terminus, which can also be done with the patient lying facedown.

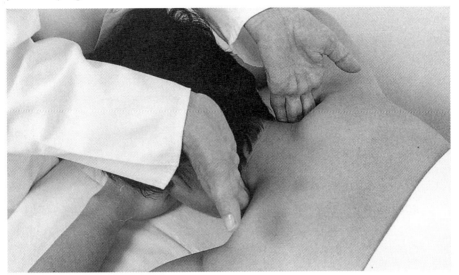

THE LYMPHATIC SYSTEM HANDBOOK

TREATMENT OF THE OCCIPITAL REGION

This treatment, called the *pyramid*, is very useful for headaches caused by nervous tension, high blood pressure, and neck pain.

1. The treatment consists of pushing the lymph downward and outward with all the fingertips placed along the nape of the neck, following a line that should be as long as the distance between the mastoids (the bony protuberances behind the ears). In a second stage, the fingers move upwards, reducing their line of support and moving closer together.

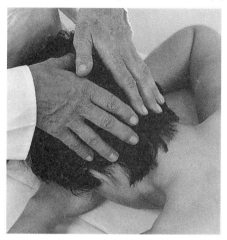
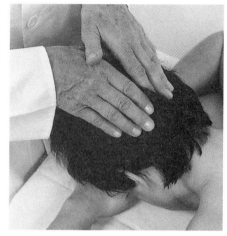

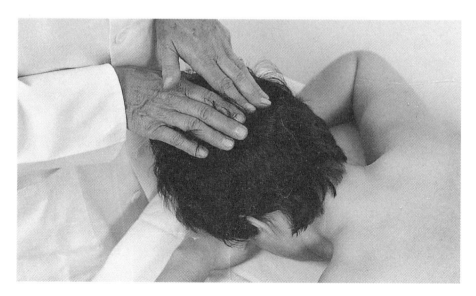

2. At the apex of the cranial vault, the therapist places the palm of the hand and presses in a semicircular movement ("closing the pyramid").

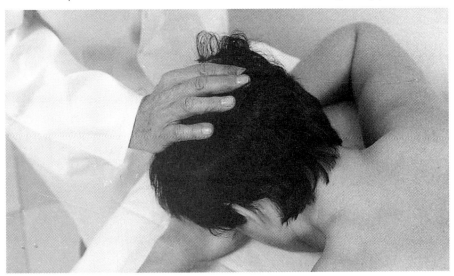

3. The posterior auricular lymph nodes are then emptied, where the lymph from the occipital region has arrived after the pyramid has been executed.

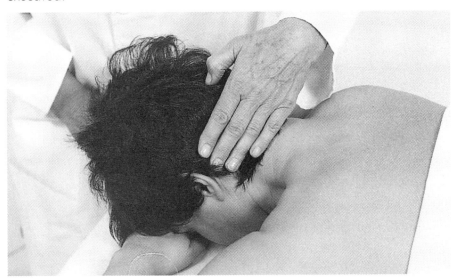

4. Pressure is applied on the posterior auricular lymph nodes to pump the lymph downward. This is done first on one side and then on the other.

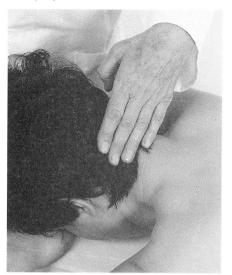 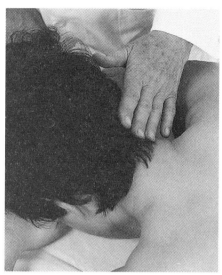

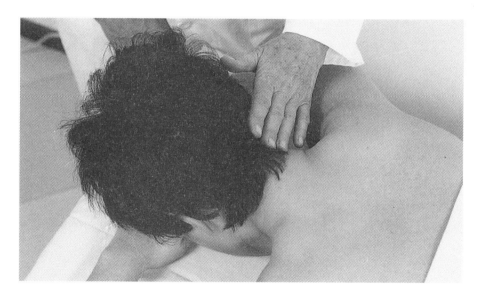

5. The profundus (the lower auricular lymph nodes) and finally the terminus are treated (see the phases in photographs 16 and 17 on pages 96–97.

TREATMENT OF THE OCCIPITAL AND CERVICAL REGION

This is a very useful treatment in cases of headaches located in the frontal and posteroinferior (occipital) part of the skull, as well as in pain caused by hypertension, cervical stiffness, cervical arthrosis, and torticollis (wryneck).

1. It starts with a pumping technique known as *pomper-renvoier* ("pumping-sending"), the main movement of which is very similar to the action of sweeping the floor, as it involves pushing and concentrating excess lymph in one spot and then collecting it. In this case, one hand alternatively pushes and the other one collects, precipitating the lymph toward the cervical region.

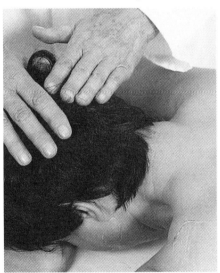 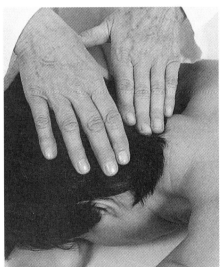

2. The lymph from the cervical region is then pushed toward the para-vertebral lymph nodes, which are located along the cervical spine. In this way, using semicircular movements, pressure is applied to the spine. The fingertips should be placed on top of the vertebrae (median posterior part) but without touching them.

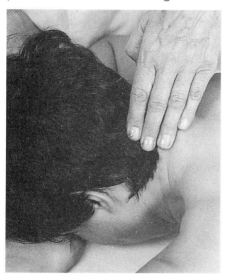 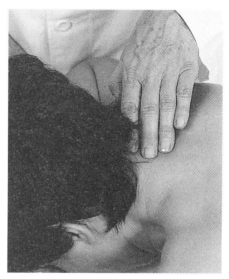

3. With open hands, push on top of the deltoids toward the terminus.

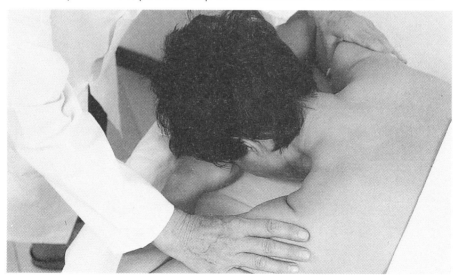

4. The lymph is then pushed from the upper trapezius (shoulder line) toward the terminus.

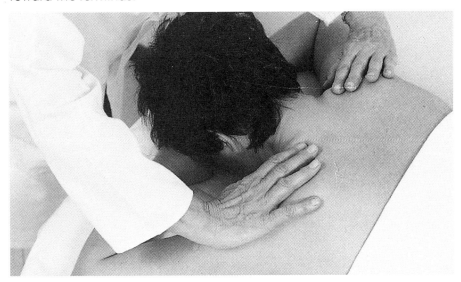

5. Finally, place the fingers at the same height as the nuchal line and vibrate them slightly to make a slight traction on the spine for two seconds. Rest for a further two seconds and repeat the operation about five times.

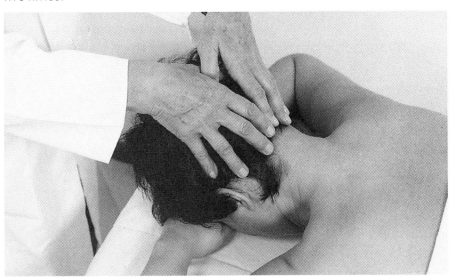

TREATMENT OF THE ARM

This treatment is very useful in treating and curing shoulder pain, epicondylitis, epitrochleitis, omoplato-humeral periarthritis, carpal tunnel syndrome, tingling, paresthesia in the hands (alterations in sensitivity), wrist distensions, trauma, fractures, and other symptoms.

1. Start with the deltoid muscle. The right hand performs the drainage and the left hand holds the arm.

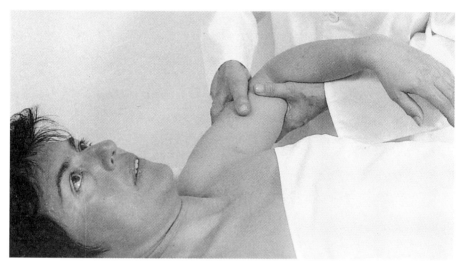

2. The right hand is then moved to the upper part of the deltoid.

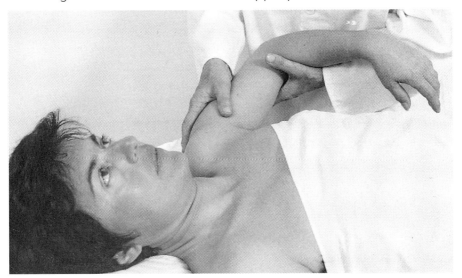

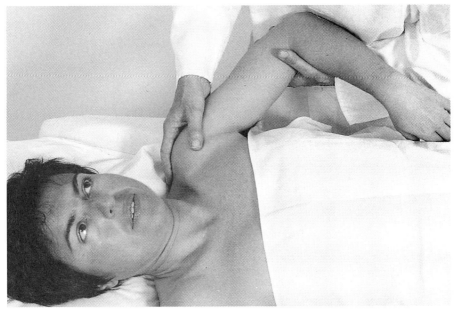

3. With light pressure, the lymph from the arm is sent to the axillary lymph nodes.

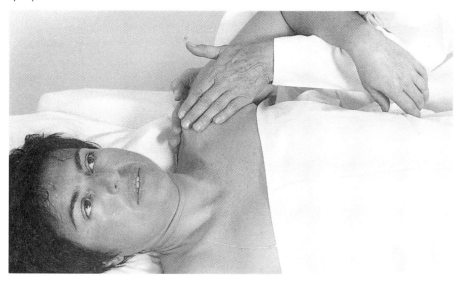

4. The axillary lymph nodes are emptied by pressing with the fingers, except for the thumbs.

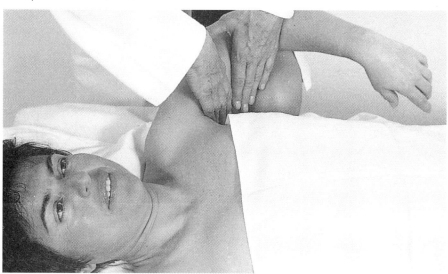

5. The axillary emptying is performed: one hand is placed under the shoulder and moved slightly while the other hand pushes over the axillary lymph nodes toward the terminus.

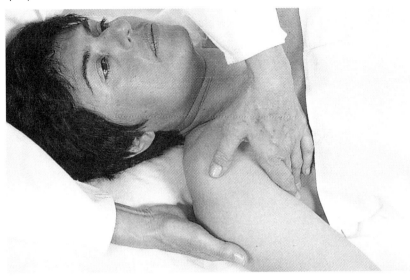

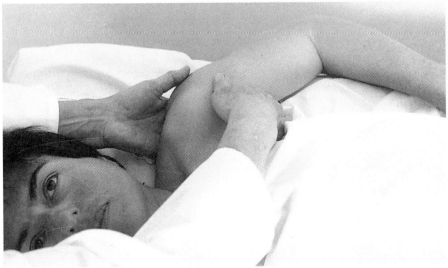

6. Drainage of the epicondyle and epitrochlea at the elbow is continued. To do this, one hand holds the upper arm and the other moves in a spiral motion over the epicondyle and epitrochlea (the outer and inner bony parts of the elbow). This manipulation is particularly useful in cases of epicondylitis and epitrochleitis.

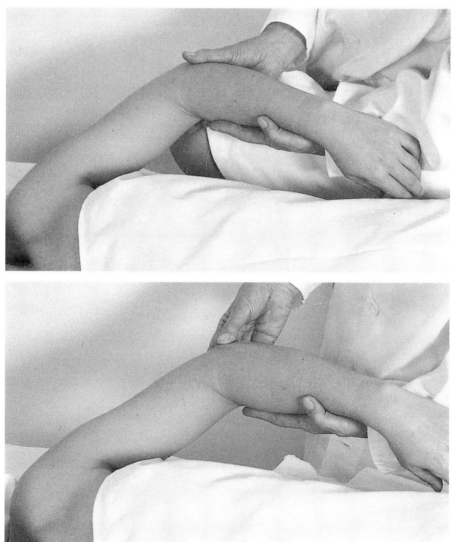

7. The ulnar lymph nodes are emptied with the thumb, placed in the crease of the elbow.

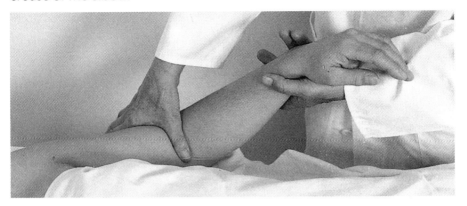

8. Then pump with the palm of one hand from the dorsal part of the forearm while the other hand is directed toward the armpit, to promote lymphatic flow.

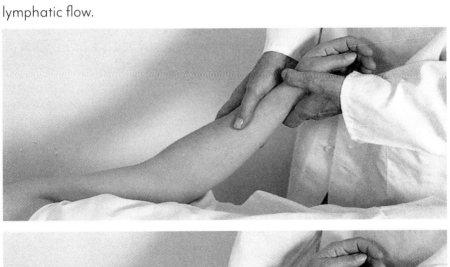

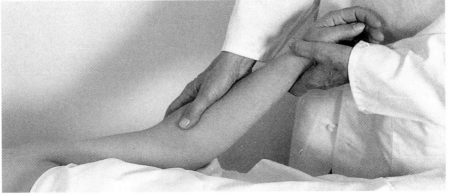

9. The inside of the forearm is pumped, from the wrist to the lymph nodes at the elbow.

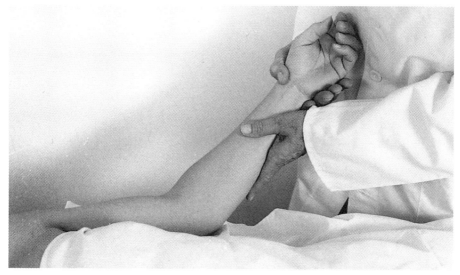

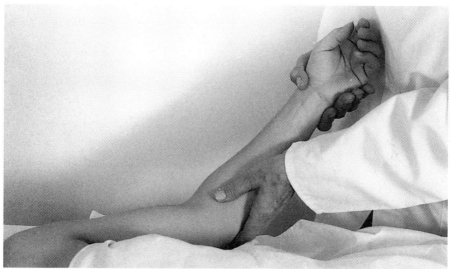

10. The wrist is drained by alternating pushes of the two thumbs.

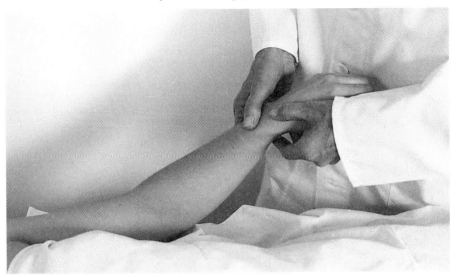

11. The palm of the hand is treated with light spiral pressure. All fingers except the thumbs are used for this.

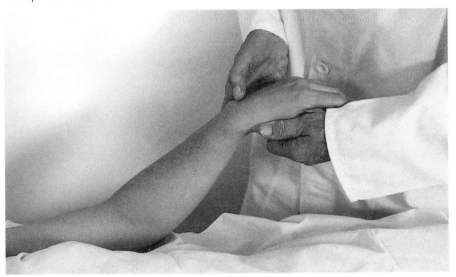

12. Next, the interosseous spaces on the back of the hand are drained. To do this, spiral movements should be made with the thumb from the heads of the metacarpals to the wrist. In the meantime, the other hand will support the arm. This treatment is very useful after trauma or paralysis, or in cases of arthrosis or motor disorders.

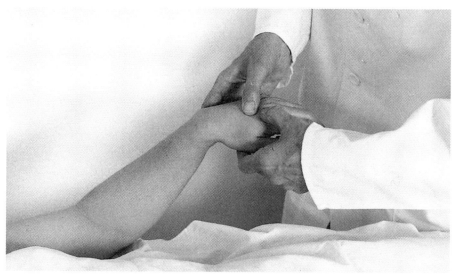

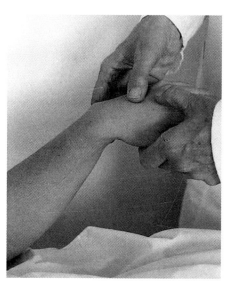

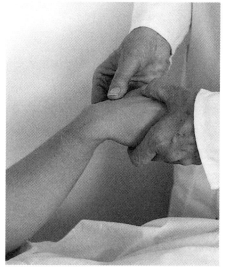

13. The treatment of the index, middle, ring, and little fingers is carried out by means of small pressures with the thumbs, from the tip to the base of each finger. The massage should be done alternately: first the index finger, then the ring finger, then the middle finger, and finally the little finger.

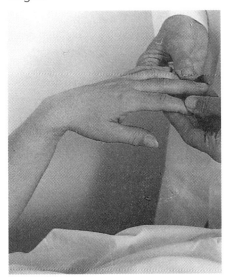 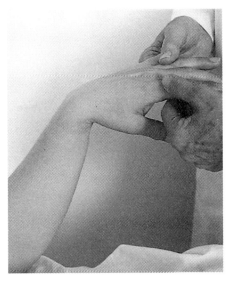

14. Last, the palm of the hand and the thenar eminence (muscle located on the fifth metacarpal bone that allows thumb movements) are massaged. The therapist's two thumbs are moved alternately in small spiral semicircles.

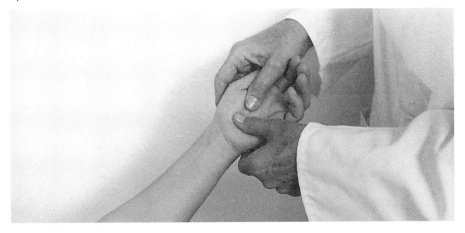

LYMPHATIC DRAINAGE OF THE BREAST

This treatment can help to prevent breast diseases, in particular fibro-cystic mastopathy (small nodules in the breast), cysts, tumors, and aesthetisms caused by the weakening of the supporting tissues.

1. Through a squeezing movement, the lymph moves from the base of the breast toward the areola.

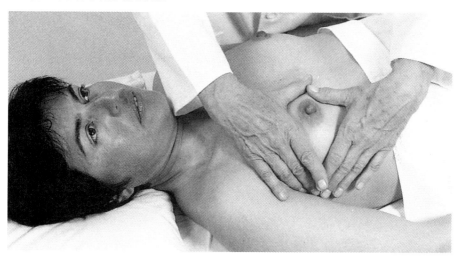

2. While immobilizing the areola with one hand, push on the axillary lymph nodes with the other hand.

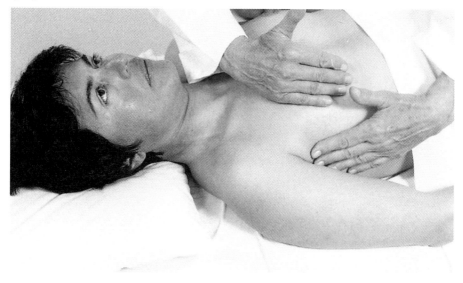

3. Finally, the axillary lymph nodes are emptied.

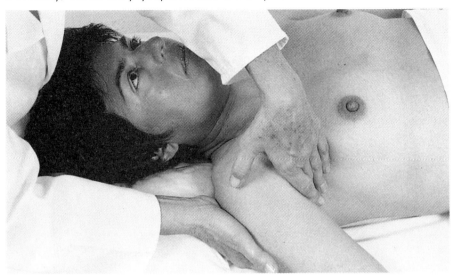

THE **LYMPHATIC SYSTEM HANDBOOK**

LYMPHATIC DRAINAGE OF THE THORAX

This treatment also completes the drainage of the breast, improving the circulation of lymph at the level of the thorax. It is useful in all respiratory conditions, especially in cases of chronic bronchitis and pleurisy, as well as trauma to the thorax, which prevents full movement of the rib cage during breathing.

1. Apply both hands and start pumping by moving them alternately, so that one hand pushes the lymph and the other collects it in the later costal region, under the armpit.

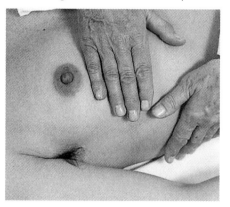 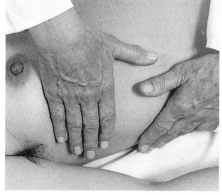

2. The lymph is directed toward the axilla. In these two phases, the lymph is pushed deeply along the intercostal spaces (and from there into the thoracic duct) with the fingers of the hand that performs the movement—in this case, the right hand, whose fingers rest on the intercostal spaces.

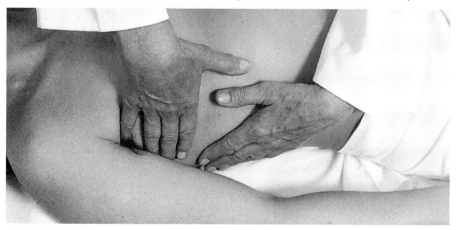

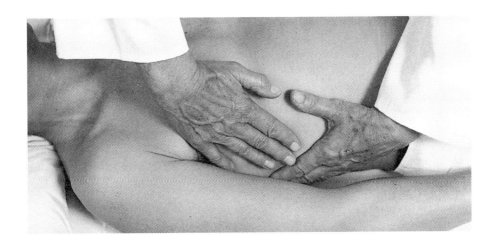

LYMPHATIC DRAINAGE OF THE ABDOMEN

This is useful for reducing cellulite on the hips and abdomen, but also to help overcome constipation by treating the descending (left) and ascending (right) colon.

1. To begin, one hand is placed on the left side, on the ileum (the upper part of the hips), while the other, placed on top of the first, performs some pumping movements. The lymph thus moves upward until it reaches the iliac crest.

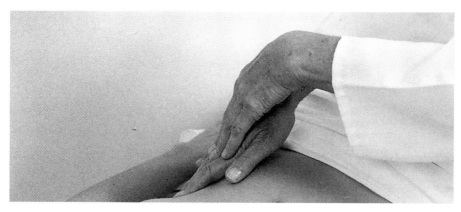

2. From the iliac crest, the lymph is brought down toward the inguinal lymph nodes, following the course of the terminal part of the left colon, the sigma, and the rectum.

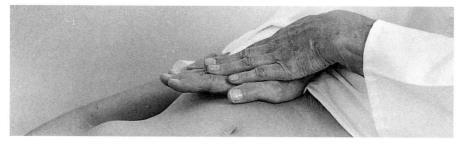

3. On the ascending colon the same movement is performed.

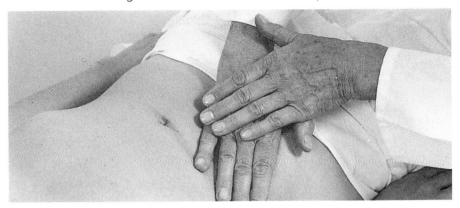

4. The right flexure of the transverse colon continues to be acted upon.

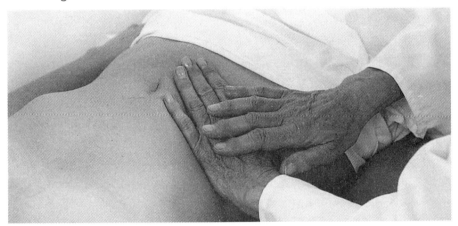

5. By a spiral movement of the hand on the descending colon, the intestinal transit is relieved and promoted.

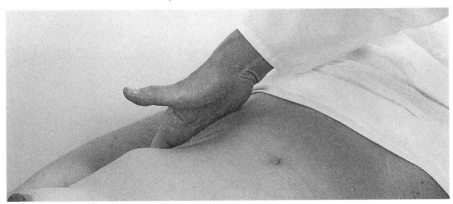

6. Support the outside of the index finger and turn the hand until all fingers are fully supported. This breaks up any fecal residues and promotes their elimination.

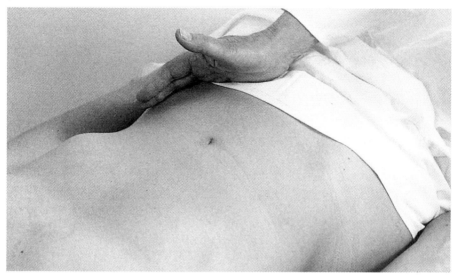

7. Next, the ascending colon is massaged with the pads of the thumbs. With a pushing movement in a semicircle, the lymph is moved and the ascending colon is stimulated to promote the elimination of feces.

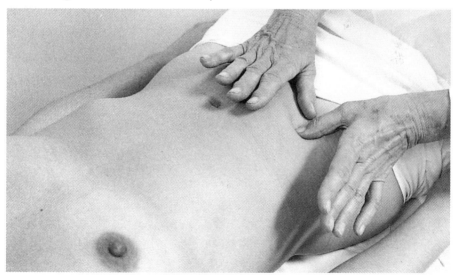

8. Finally, the iliac lymph nodes, located below the iliac crest, are emptied. The lymph is pushed deep into the iliac crest, where it is collected by the iliac ducts and sent to Pecquet's cistern.

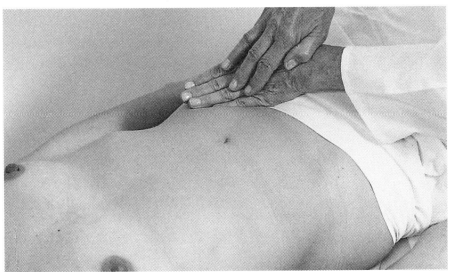

TREATMENT OF THE SCAPULA

This massage is useful for treating omoplatohumeral periarthritis as well as back pain.

1. With the fingertips, the lymph is pushed toward the inner margin of the scapula using semicircular movements to empty the lymph nodes in this area.

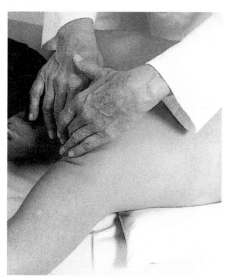
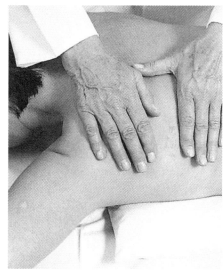
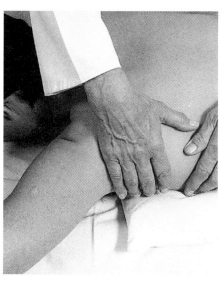
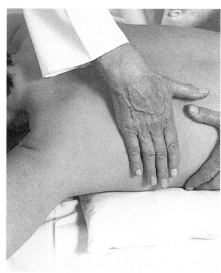

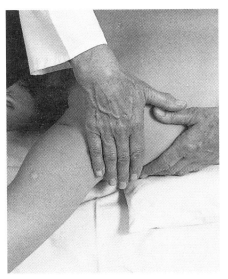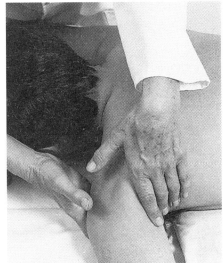

TREATMENT OF THE DORSAL AND LUMBAR SPINE

This treatment offers advantageous results for any spinal pain, osteoarthritis, trauma, stiffness, or muscle contraction.

1. The lymph accumulated on the sides of the spine is pushed with the fingertips toward the inside, where the paravertebral lymph nodes are located, and from there to the thoracic duct.

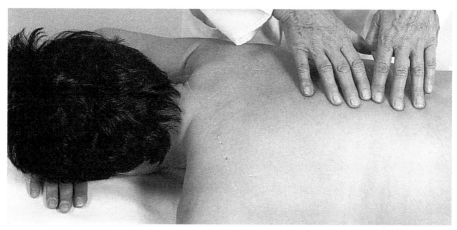

2. When manipulating the dorsal region, the fingertips of the index, middle, and ring fingers are placed in the center of the back and massaged so that the lymph flows inward until it almost reaches the thorax.

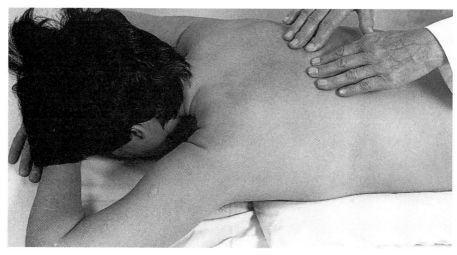

3. Repeat the same operation on the lumbar area.

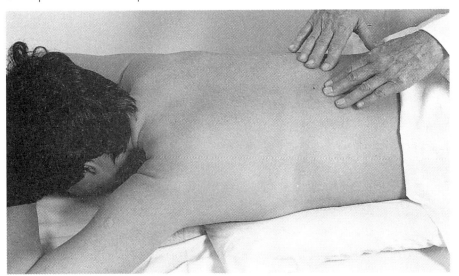

THE **LYMPHATIC SYSTEM HANDBOOK**

TREATMENT OF THE SACRAL AND BUTTOCK REGION

This treatment is useful for all sacral and lumbosacral pain, herniated discs in the last lumbar vertebrae, sciatica, and osteoarthritis of the hip (coxitis) and the lumbosacral area, as well as cellulitis and coccyx pain.

1. To empty the lymph from the subcutis of the lumbosacral region and the buttocks, push with the palms of the hands toward the upper part of the buttocks. Then repeat the same operation from the sacrum to the middle part and finally from the same point to the lower part.

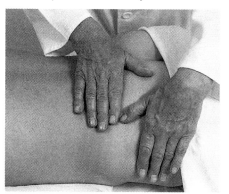 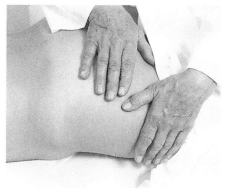

2. The following movement allows the lymph nodes located in the musculature of the lumbosacral region, buttocks, and coccyx to be emptied. For this, the previous treatment is repeated from the sacroiliac region. To begin with, an almost horizontal line is followed, whereas in the following steps, when the lymph is pushed from the sacrum toward the coccyx and the perineum, the route will be more vertical. In this case, the drainage, instead of being done with the palms, will be carried out with the fingertips of one hand, on which you will place the other hand to give more strength to your push.

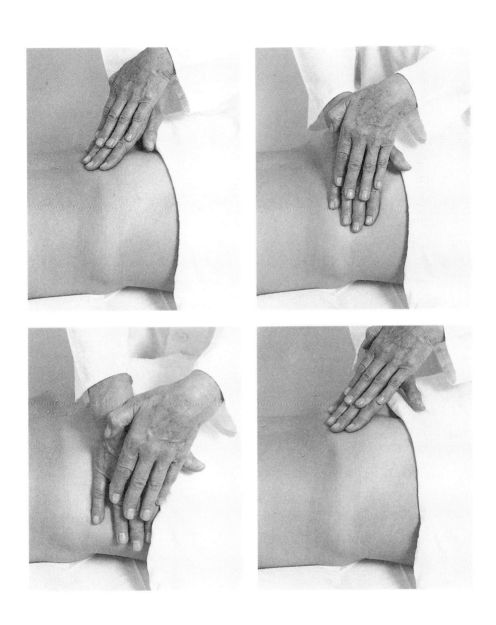

THE LYMPHATIC SYSTEM HANDBOOK

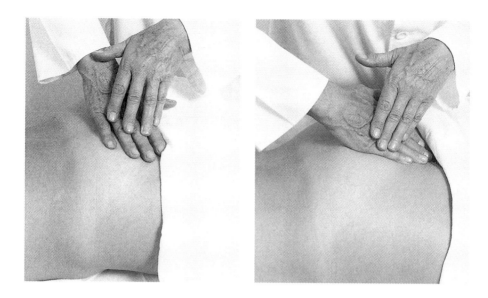

3. Finally, the iliac lymph nodes are discharged, from which the lymph reaches the inguinal lymph nodes and, in part, goes directly into the deep iliac ducts, which are tributaries of Pecquet's cistern.

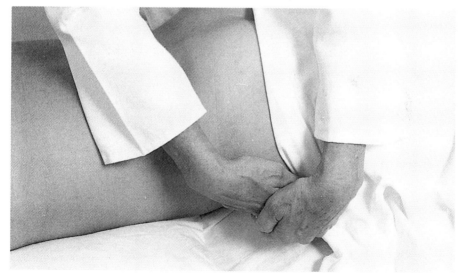

TREATMENT OF THE THIGHS

This treatment is useful for venous insufficiency, cellulite, thigh pain, sciatica, cramps, and lactic acid buildup after exercise. It is often useful in sports medicine as well.

1. The patient should be positioned on the back. The therapist will place one hand above and one hand below the thigh and begin to move them alternately in several semicircles. In this way, the lymph in the medial and lateral areas of the thigh is pushed.

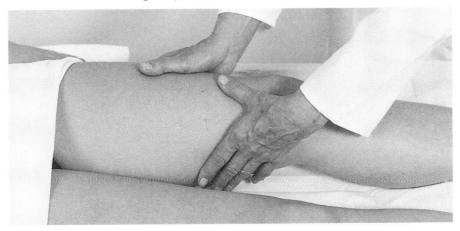

2. In this way, the hand placed on the lateral surface reaches the upper thigh, while the other hand continues to push the lymph down the medial side.

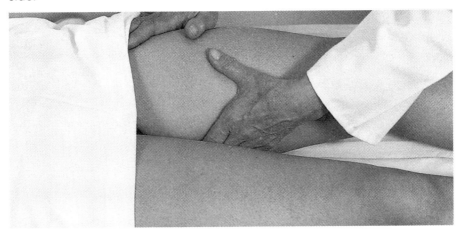

3. Place the hands side by side in a flat position and press gently with the fingertips on the lymph nodes of the abductor muscles, thus emptying them.

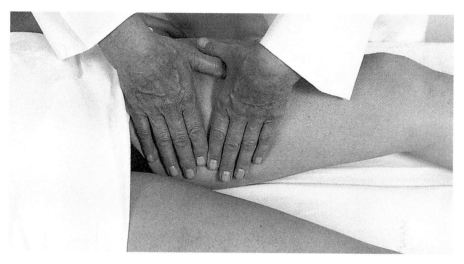

4. The inguinal lymph nodes are then emptied. The hand that previously worked on the outside is placed on top of the groin to perform a light, rhythmic pumping of the inguinal lymph nodes. This pushes the lymph toward the iliac ducts, which collect the lymph from the legs and pelvis and then make it flow toward Pecquet's cistern. The other hand, placed on top of the first, assists in the action, simultaneously making a light, rhythmic thrust.

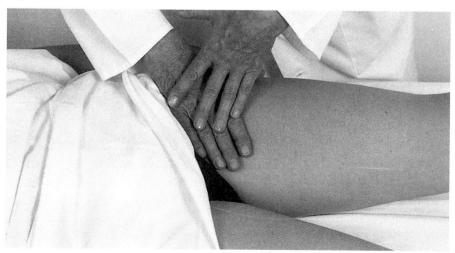

5. Then, using the pump-and-send technique (see page 119), the lymph is "collected" and sent out again. The hand furthest back does the pumping.

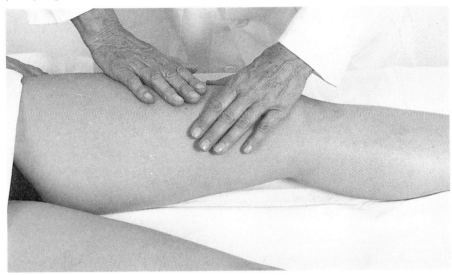

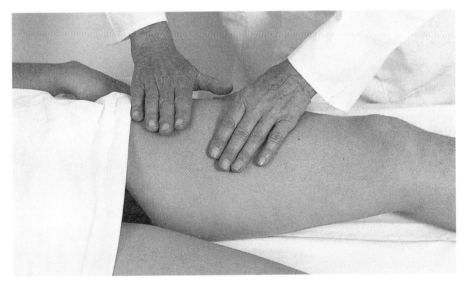

6. The third step consists of a deep hollowing of the thigh with the palms of the hands and the fingertips. One hand is placed on the inside and the other on the outside of the thigh, and the upper part of the thigh is then "hollowed out," near the beginning of the thigh. Then move to the middle area and finally work above the knee. The drainage technique used is called the bracelet technique, as the hands and fingertips push at the same time toward the beginning of the thigh and squeeze it. The fingertips, placed behind the thigh, empty the posterior lymph nodes.

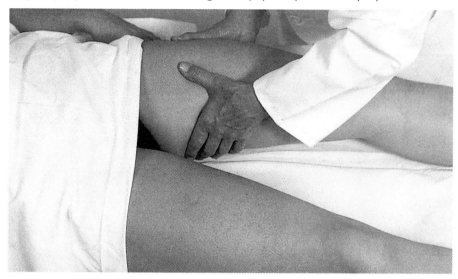

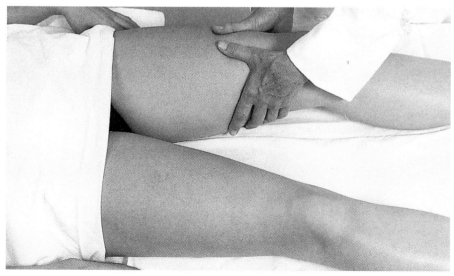

7. With the patient facedown, move both hands in semicircles alternately. One hand pushes with palm and thumb upward and toward the inner surface of the thigh, while the other pushes toward the outer surface of the thigh, allowing the physiological drainage of lymph.

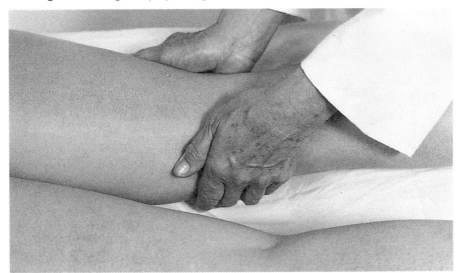

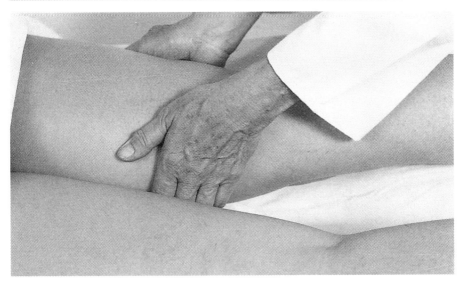

8. Finally, the popliteal lymph nodes are emptied.

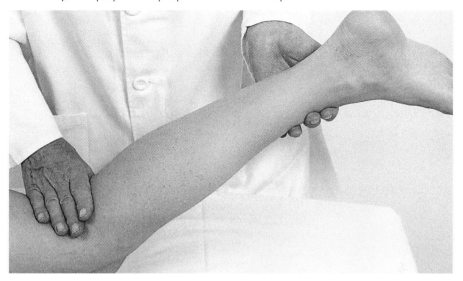

TREATMENT OF THE KNEE

This treatment is useful for the prevention of osteoarthritis of the knee as well as for the treatment of trauma to the bony parts of the joint (fractures of the tibia, femur, or fibula), and also for the ligaments and tendons of the knee. In addition, it is useful in the treatment of meniscus injuries and the reeducation of mobility after a long period of immobilization. Finally, localized lymphatic drainage helps to eliminate cellulite in the knee.

1. Above the median part of the knee, a gentle pumping movement is performed (see page 119): the upper hand picks up the lymph and the other hand, placed underneath, pushes it toward the lymph nodes at the back of the knee.

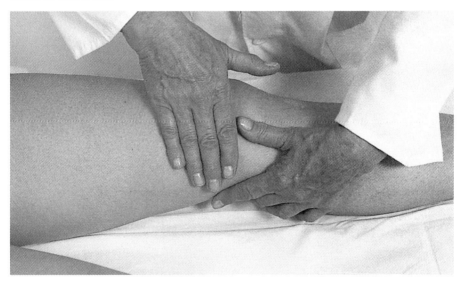

2. The hands, with the fingers extended, push deep and upwards; in this way, the lymph will be directed toward the lymph nodes at the back of the knee and will continue its superficial course in the anterior and medial part of the thigh.

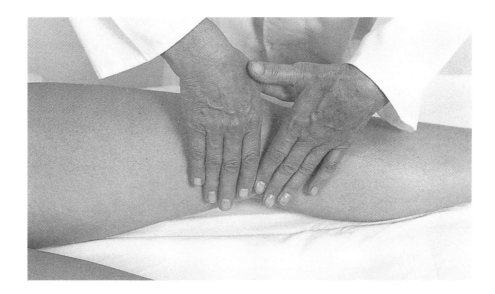

3. The popliteal cavity (back of the knee) is then emptied with the fingertips, which are pushed in deeply. To do this, the therapist places one of the wrists on the bed and lifts the joint slightly with the fingers.

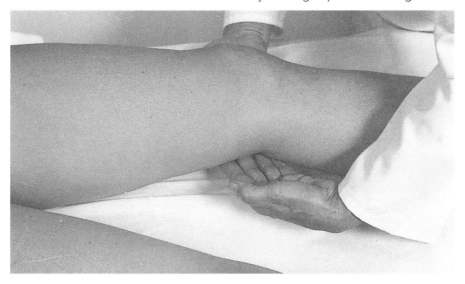

4. The patella is then massaged from bottom to top with the palm of one hand, while the other hand continues to press on the popliteal cavity.

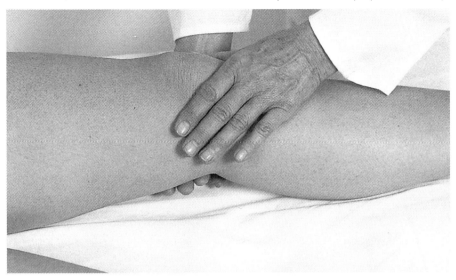

5. The thenar eminence of the hand and the thumbs are pushed inward over the margins of the patella to empty the corresponding lymph nodes, first those at the top and then those at the bottom.

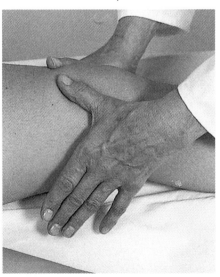
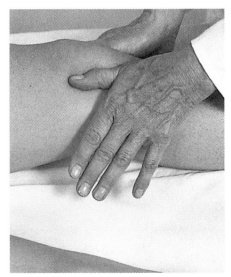

6. Bring the fingertips together near the tibial protuberance. Keeping their position and always practicing a semicircular movement, gently push upward toward the inguinal lymph nodes.

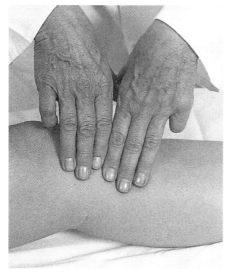 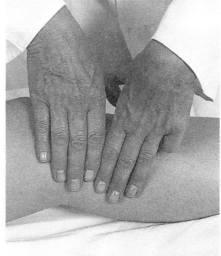

KNEE SWELLING IN ADOLESCENTS

Lymphatic drainage of the knee is very useful in relieving swellings, especially those caused by too-rapid growth during adolescence. The treatment explained in these pages has been used to cure a swelling caused by cartilage inflammation in an eleven-year-old boy. The manipulations are the same as those described above.

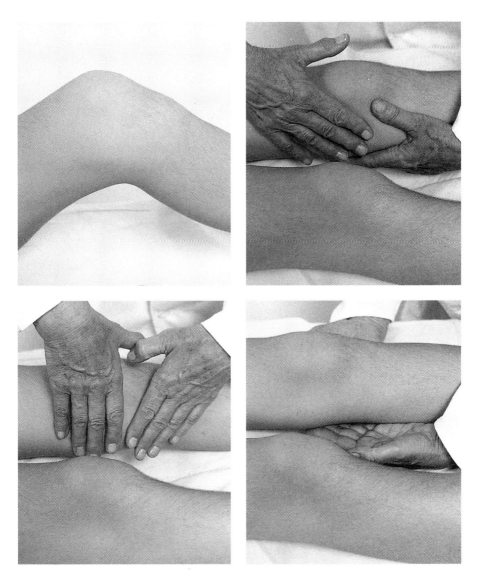

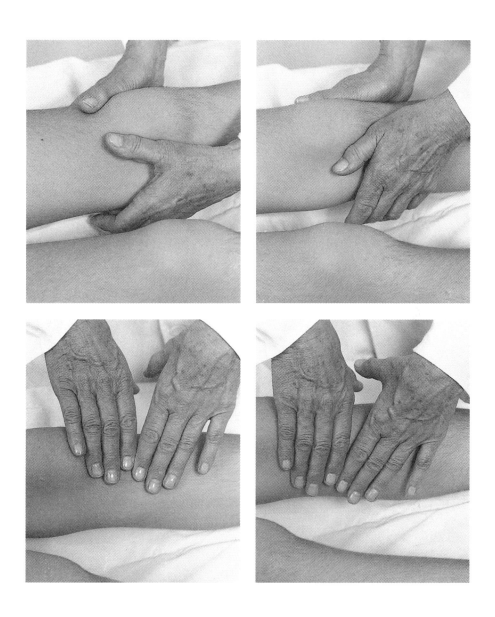

LEG TREATMENT

This treatment is very suitable for venous insufficiency of the legs, cellulite, and cramps.

1. The patient is placed on the back. The therapist places his hands below the knee and massages rhythmically up the back of the leg.

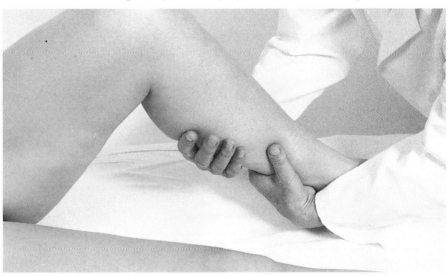

2. Drainage is then carried out in the usual manner.

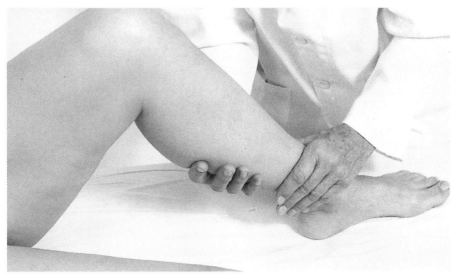

3. With the patient now lying facedown, a two-handed drainage is performed on the back of the leg. One hand is placed higher than the other so that all the lymph is directed into the popliteal cavity.

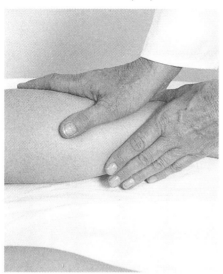 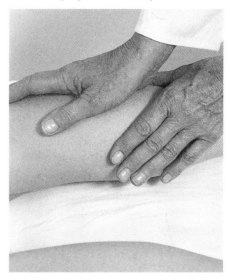

4. Next, the lower part of the calf is pumped.

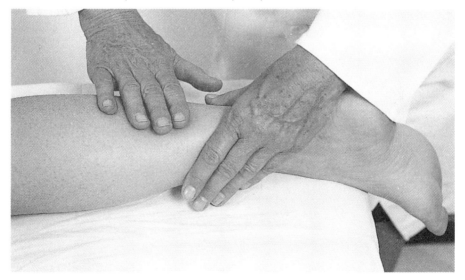

5. Finally, the whole process is repeated on the middle and upper parts of the calf.

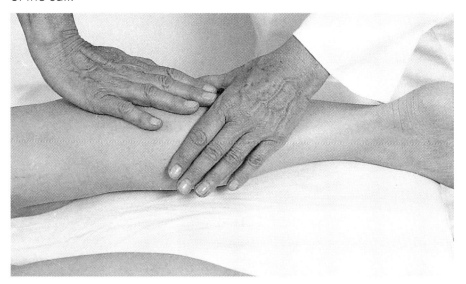

ACHILLES TENDON TREATMENT

This treatment is very useful in cases of venous insufficiency of the leg, cellulitis, tendonitis, heel inflammations, and foot-support defects.

1. With the patient on the back, one of the therapist's hands lifts the foot while the other drains the tendon. The treatment is carried out with the fingertips, the thumb on one side and the remaining fingers on the other. From the heel, they move upward with a rhythmic movement and a push.

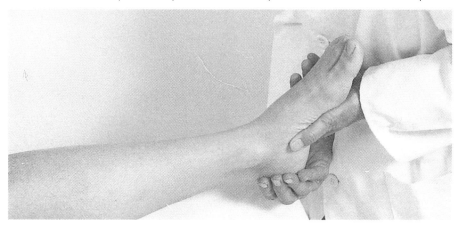

2. With the patient facedown, the same treatment is repeated: first, the Achilles heel is massaged from below and then from above.

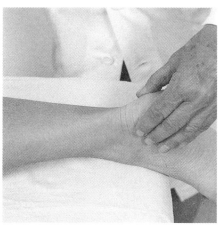 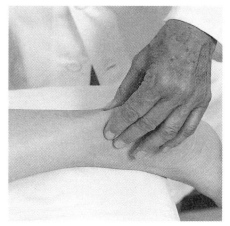

TREATMENT OF THE ANKLE AND MALLEOLI

This treatment is useful for ankle strains and sprains, for the reeducation of mobility after ankle and malleolus injuries, in cases of venous insufficiency of the legs, and finally to treat cellulite.

1. Massage the anterior part of the malleoli with the fingers, except the thumbs. One hand is placed on each part. The fingertips always make the same semicircular thrust, in the posterior direction and above.

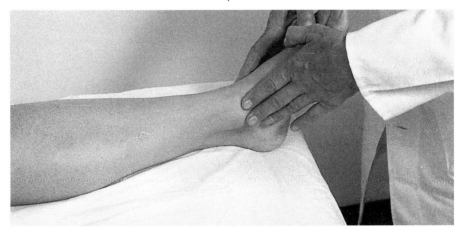

2. A similar procedure is followed by pushing from the back upward.

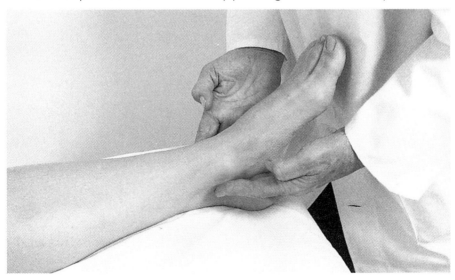

TREATMENT OF THE DORSUM AND INSTEP OF THE FOOT

This treatment is useful for all foot and ankle complaints, venous insufficiency, and cellulite of the legs.

1. The fingers (except the thumbs) are pushed upward rhythmically in a semicircular direction with the fingers together.

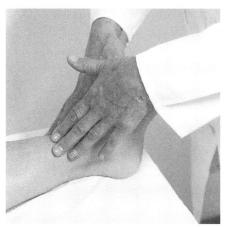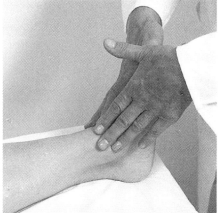

TREATMENT OF THE INTEROSSEOUS SPACES OF THE FOOT

This treatment is useful for all foot complaints, support defects, cramps in the feet and toes, ankle trauma, and the like.

1. The lymph is pushed upward (in the direction of the ankle) with the pads of the thumbs, alternately, while making semicircular movements.

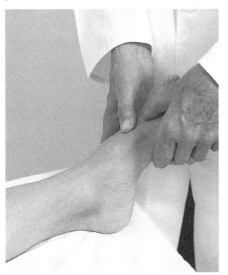 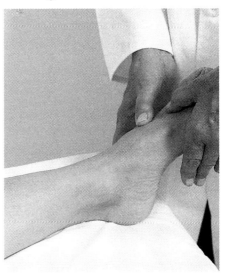

TREATMENT OF THE HALLUX (BIG TOE)

This treatment relieves all foot support problems and helps in cases of acute pain, especially metatarsal pain.

1. The toe is pinched between the thenar eminence and the therapist's thumb and squeezed gently but firmly.

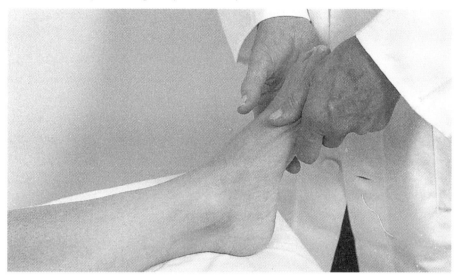

TREATMENT OF THE TOES, EXCEPT THE HALLUX (BIG TOE)

This treatment is useful in cases of swollen ankles, acute metatarsal pain, and foot movement recovery therapies.

1. Simultaneous pressure is applied to the second and fourth toes, changing the point of application and proceeding from the extremity toward the base of each toe.

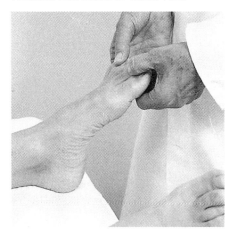 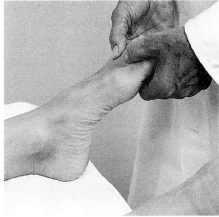

2. The same operation should be done with the third and fourth fingers.

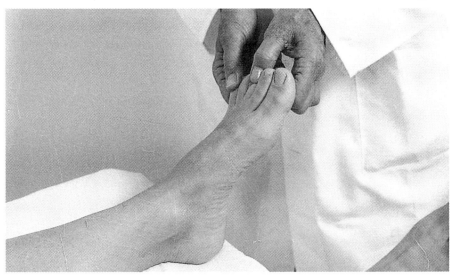

TREATMENT OF THE TARSUS

This treatment is useful in relieving metatarsalgia (metatarsal pain), foot support defects, swelling of the ankles, and venous insufficiency of the legs.

1. The foot is grasped with both hands and squeezed, starting at the extremity and working up to the ankle.

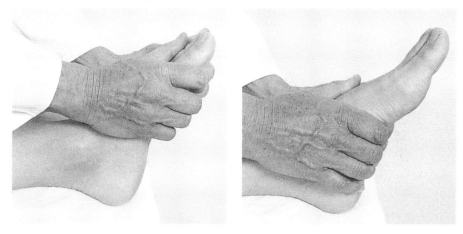

Chapter 7

LYMPHATIC CIRCULATION AND WELL-BEING

THE SEVEN MAIN RULES

When a person is tired, she should rest; when she is sleepy, she should sleep; when she needs to go to the toilet, she should go.

In everyday life and especially at work, it is normal that these basic rules cannot be followed. However, the lymphatic circulation works well when you live a leisurely life. The following rules must be observed:

- ensure proper nutrition;
- respect the body's needs (rest, sleep, physiological functions, and so on);
- engage in moderate physical activity;
- make time for meditation, contemplation, art, and culture;
- maintain a good family relationship;
- take part in enjoyable social activities (friendships, associations, and others);
- maintain satisfactory sexual activity.

It is therefore necessary to analyze and ask oneself a few questions about one's habits and try to correct them as much as possible. This is often less difficult than one might think.

FOOD

Waste products produced by improper nutrition can often be deposited in the lymphatic system. Excessive accumulation leads to lymphatic stasis and disease.

The ideal daily diet should avoid fats, fried foods, sweets, alcoholic beverages, sausages, milk (replace with yogurt), chocolate, sweet drinks, and also should limit the consumption of tea, coffee, and chamomile tea as much as possible. However, once a week you can eat whatever you like.

For the body to function properly, the combination of grains (bread, pasta, rice, and so forth) with protein foods (meat, cheese, eggs, nuts, seeds, legumes, fish, and the like) in a single meal should be avoided.

It is also important to vary the diet, changing the type of grains and the type of protein food each day. Even vegetables, which can accompany one or the other, should be varied.

Eat calmly, chewing each mouthful well and avoiding talking about unpleasant things while eating. In addition to favoring the digestive processes, the food thus introduced into the body will be better assimilated, and above all the eater will be satisfied with smaller quantities, without overloading the stomach with excessive food.

In this regard, it makes no sense to impose diets that drastically limit food intake: if a person is hungry, he or she should eat, and if thirsty, should drink. If a person eats and drinks too much, dietary errors and excesses should be corrected.

Little salting, sweetening, and seasoning allows the taste of food to be appreciated and prepares the stomach for digestion. In fact, well-chewed food produces chemical and nerve signals that correctly inform the stomach and the other organs of digestion about the level of acidity and the amount of enzymes needed for digestion.

On the other hand, too much salt accentuates the desire to drink more, which causes excessive dilution of the gastric, duodenal, and pancreatic juices necessary for digestion, reducing its effectiveness. The same applies to sugar and condiments in general.

If a person gets into the habit of salting, sweetening, and seasoning little of what she eats, she will digest better and, above all, will soon eat only the amount of food necessary to live.

Finally, do not underestimate the positive effect that two words of thanks to God or to Nature, as well as to the person who prepared the meal, have at the beginning of a meal. This is a reflection that helps us to be aware of the importance of the food that enriches the very act of eating.

THE DREAM

The night's sleep may not have been enough, perhaps because of a bad habit of spending the whole night in front of the TV or smartphone, or going to bed late.

To avoid tiredness and drowsiness during the day, you should not spend too much time watching television, but only use it when you are looking for something specific, and try to set a maximum time. If the broadcast you are interested in ends too late, you can record it on video and watch it the next day.

Daytime sleepiness can sometimes be dependent on nighttime insomnia. Drowsiness, in turn, has two main causes, which can occur simultaneously: poor digestion and worry.

To remedy poor digestion, it is necessary to reread and perhaps put into practice the principles outlined in the previous paragraph on nutrition.

Worries are negative emotions, unprocessed during the day, that come back to occupy our heads at night, blocking serene rest. Get used to meditating before bed and think aloud again about what happened during the day, expressing good intentions and plans to solve the problems that arose. Finally, we need to trust in our own goodwill, as well as in that of God or Nature, which harmonizes everything.

PHYSIOLOGICAL NEEDS

According to traditional Chinese medicine, bile function is active between 11 p.m. and 1 a.m., liver function between 1 a.m. and 3 a.m., lung function between 3 a.m. and 5 a.m., and colon function between 5 a.m. and 7 a.m. When the colon is active, its activity, which is to prepare the output of feces, ends at 7 a.m., that would be the best time to go to the toilet. It is important, in order to give the right rhythm to the bowel, to get uscd to regularity, even if the first few times you do not notice a particular need. After a few days, the bowel will get used to it and will function regularly, which, in addition to being in harmony with the body's other rhythms, will avoid one's having to go to the toilet during the day, something that is not always possible. Many people, in fact, suffer from constipation because too often, in order not to interrupt their work or other activities, they ignore the stimuli of the bowel, which adapts even to bad habits. Constipation in turn leads to intoxication of the organism as well as lymphatic stasis. It is also a mistake to prevent urination: during the day we should get used to emptying our bladder every two hours, even when we do not notice the stimulus.

PHYSICAL AND MANUAL ACTIVITY, MEDITATION, SOCIAL LIFE, AND SEXUALITY

Movement is important, if possible done outdoors or in a gym or even at home, so as to maintain elasticity and a satisfactory relationship with the world.

Time spent in meditation, art, and culture is not time wasted; quite the contrary. It is essential to nourish our mental and spiritual needs; doing so enables us to have new ideas every day and to escape from stereotypes. It also promotes a more balanced state of mind, which helps all bodily functions, including lymphatic circulation.

Concerning the relationship between body and mind, it is necessary to underline the importance of having good dialogue in the family, which too often is forgotten under the pretext of following the rhythms of everyday life. Try to find some time to share with your relatives: talking with them, asking questions, and laughing all provide important psychic as well as spiritual nourishment.

It is good to talk to friends and, if possible, to meet them in person now and then. Sometimes a phone call is enough to share pleasant emotions. Our psyche and our body will both be grateful for this good habit.

We need to put the above points into practice, so as to get back to enjoying pleasant and natural sex. The harmony created around us then acts as an accumulator that keeps our "batteries" always charged. Sex then becomes a ritual that celebrates the couple, moving the kundalini energy from the spiritual center of the seventh chakra (cusp of the head), through the spine, to the first chakra in the genital area.[7]

---

7 According to Indian medicine, the chakras are seven centers in our body that receive, transform, and emit energy. The energy and life force that run through our body are called *kundalini*.

Chapter 8

CELLULITE

GENERAL

Cellulite is commonly understood as an infiltration and stagnation of water and fat in the subcutaneous tissues. It tends to occur more frequently in women than in men, especially on the thighs and buttocks, and is usually due to hormonal causes. In fact, the female cycle requires that water and nutrients are regularly brought to the pelvis, which are necessary for the uterus, so that, in the event of fertilization, the embryo can be in the best conditions for its survival and development.

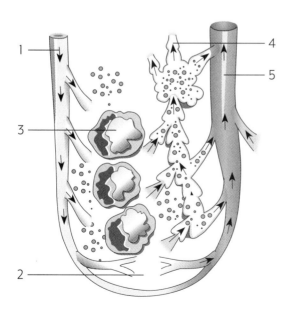

Normal arterial, venous, and lymphatic circulatory status

1. Artery
2. Capillaries
3. Adipose cell
4. Lymphatic vessels
5. Vein

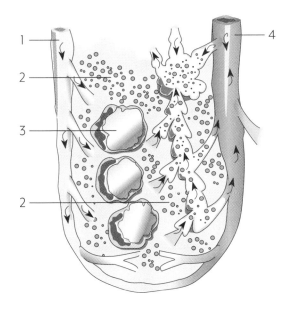

This pathological condition is caused by venous and lymphatic circulatory reduction. Veins and lymphatic vessels have dilated, fat has accumulated inside the cell, and fluids have stagnated.

1. Artery
2. Edema
3. Adipose cell
4. Vein

Cellulitis is caused by lymphatic and venous stasis. The initial, intermediate, and final degenerative phases of the skin and subcutaneous tissue are shown here.

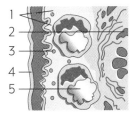
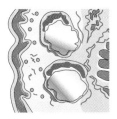
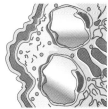

1. Fluids
2. Capillaries
3. Fibrous tissue
4. Cutis
5. Adipose

In the initial phase of lymphatic stasis, fluids begin to stagnate in the tissues, which is why fat cells are unable to expel fat.

As the fluids remain stagnant, the accumulation of fat causes a loosening of the complexion and, by reaction, the formation of fibrous tissue.

As cells increase, the capillaries break down and fibrous tissue takes up the entire space.

In the absence of fertilization, the accumulated fluids are removed partly by menstruation and partly via the regional lymphatic vessels. These vessels are mainly connected to the inguinal lymph nodes and to the genital hypogastric lymph nodes, from which the iliac lymphatic duct and the hypogastric lymphatic duct, respectively, exit. The lymph then reaches Pecquet's cistern, from which the thoracic duct arises, reaching the venous circle in the left subclavian vein (see pages 37–40).

If this system is blocked at any point, fluids do not flow away completely and tend to stagnate in the thighs and buttocks and also in internal organs, favoring, for example, the formation of hemorrhoids.

There are further obstacles to the proper removal of fluids and lymph; the causes mainly relate to insufficient or irregular menstruation and a sedentary lifestyle.

CELLULITE CAUSED BY MENSTRUAL CYCLE IRREGULARITIES

The cause of delayed or insufficient menstruation that, in turn, is caused by the accumulation of cellulitis, must always be sought in the reduced functional activity of the ovaries, which can be hindered by the intestine. In fact, inflammatory bowel problems on the right side, especially in the cecum[8] and appendix, act by proximity on the right ovary. Irregular functioning of the left ovary, by contrast, is often due to constipation.

Taking contraceptive pills to regulate the menstrual cycle without having resolved the bowel problems worsens the situation. It is necessary to go back and investigate the possible source of the intestinal discomfort.

The main cause is a malfunction of the digestive organs. Consequently, if there is a disturbance in digestion, substances that are not fully broken down reach the intestine and cannot be properly assim-

---

8   The cecum is the initial part of the colon, i.e., the large intestine, where the appendix is located.

ilated by the lymphatic vessels of the intestinal villi. At this point, the intestinal lymphatic vessels become clogged, causing lymphatic stasis and subsequent chronic inflammation of the intestine.

CELLULITE DUE TO A SEDENTARY LIFESTYLE

Another obstacle to the proper removal of fluids and the circulation of lymph flow is a sedentary lifestyle. Lack of muscular drive, one of the most important factors in lymph circulation, leads to lymphatic stasis or reduction.

On the other hand, sitting compresses the thighs and reduces lymph circulation. To overcome this problem, reclining chairs can be used, at least for part of the day, with the seat tilted forward so that the weight of the body is distributed between the buttocks and the knees, which rest on a padded board for this purpose. This posture avoids posterior compression of the thigh and helps to keep the spine erect, also favoring the circulation of lymph through the thoracic duct. Even the respiratory movements in this type of chair are wider and favor the drainage of lymph.

In addition, sedentary lifestyles result in lower caloric intake and an increase in adipose tissue, which moderates lymph velocity.

Finally, lack of physical activity decreases the production of digestive enzymes. In fact, the pancreas, the most important and specialized digestive organ, located in the center of the upper abdomen (between the stomach, duodenum, and bile ducts), increases its enzyme production with physical activity. This is because, with increased enzyme production, the body prepares itself to consume more food to compensate for the energy consumption due to physical activity.

CORRECTING YOUR DIET TO AVOID CELLULITE

As mentioned above, digestion influences the menstrual cycle and consequently cellulite. But why is there a disturbance in digestion? There are two main reasons: poor nutrition and psychical tension.

There are two types of remedies: dieting and fasting.

First of all, it is advisable to follow a separate diet, avoiding eating carbohydrates and proteins at the same time.

- For breakfast, yogurt can be alternated with fruit, varying each day.
- To eat one portion of raw vegetables and one portion of protein: on successive days you can alternate white meat, red meat, lean cheeses, soft-boiled eggs (yolk only), legumes, fish, and soy products.
- For dinner, have a portion of cooked vegetables and a portion of grains: alternate pasta (even stuffed pasta, just with vegetables, e.g. pumpkin), cornmeal, barley soup, oat soup, and rice.
- Drink only water.
- Avoid fats, fried foods, sweets of any kind, alcoholic beverages, cured meats, milk, and coffee.

A complete cycle of the dissociated diet lasts at least seven weeks to give noticeable effects, i.e., loss of weight and abdominal bloating, as well as recovery of the figure.

However, calorie-only diets make useless sacrifices for those with lymphatic stasis problems. In contrast, the dissociated diet does not involve any limitation on the quantity of food but is based more on the quality of food. Naturally, if this diet is always followed, the results will be even more beneficial.

Once a week, if desired, the diet can be dispensed with, perhaps in good company, when the joy aids digestion.

It is worth remembering a few basic rules: eat without rushing, instead talking about pleasant things and truly tasting the food; food should be seasoned as little as possible, to limit thirst and the consequent intake of water during meals which, by diluting digestive enzymes, slows digestion; finally, it is necessary to drink at least a liter of water between meals.

MEANS OF CELLULITE PREVENTION AND REDUCTION

In addition to these hygiene and dietary measures, what can be done to prevent, avoid, or reduce cellulite?

Here are some tips.

LYMPHATIC DRAINAGE

We have described this method, one of the best against cellulite, in detail in the chapter on lymphatic drainage (page 67). A session of lymphatic drainage, done shortly after the middle of the cycle, prevents or reduces lymphatic stagnation and is a good preventive measure.

To treat cellulite, up to two sessions per week over a long period of time may be necessary. However, the frequency and number of sessions must be determined on a case-by-case basis. In general, lymphatic drainage cannot completely get rid of the older, consolidated areas of cellulite that alter the profile of the thighs and buttocks with their unsightly orange-peel appearance. This is why lymph drainage should be practiced systematically as a preventive measure.

MESOTHERAPY

Invented in the 1960s by the French doctor Michel Pistor, mesotherapy (which literally means "targeted treatment," i.e., precisely localized) consists of undoing the typical lumps of cellulite. It uses plates (nowadays there are disposable, sterilized plates with preassembled needles) of different shapes and sizes and with a variable number of needles (between three and eighteen). By means of a syringe connected to the plate, the doctor can treat more or less extended areas, depending on the needs. The amount of fluid injected, set by the doctor, varies according to the size and severity of the lump, but is usually between 10 and 20 ml.

The pharmacological fluid used in mesotherapy is composed of enzymes, local anesthetics, and products that improve local metabolism. The enzymes break down the lump tissue so that its connective fibers, which retain water, lymphatic waste, and fat cells that form a lump, will lose consistency and thereby release the retained matter.

The local anesthetic, apart from avoiding pain, promotes local circulation and the faster removal of the residues dissolved by the enzyme preparation.

The products that complete the local action induced by the enzymes and the anesthetic are the little secret of every mesotherapist. The most common are the homeopathic ones, with no side effects, made up of various compounds and injectables, based on witch hazel, *Carduus marianus*, *Aesculus hippocastanum*, arnica, berberis, or other ingredients. They are very similar to those administered orally and cleanse the affected area while improving local metabolism and preventing the subsequent formation of cellulite.

The local injection of these homeopathic products, as they have no side effects, can be performed by the patient at home. In general, five mesotherapy sessions are sufficient to get rid of small lumps, while ten are often necessary to overcome larger and more wide-spread ones.

However, the number of sessions can be reduced if the patient also follows all the rules described above. For this purpose, it is important to understand that mesotherapy only solves the cellulite problem locally and temporarily, unless you follow a set of hygienic-dietetic, physiotherapeutic, and homeopathic measures that act on the causes.

ELECTROTHERAPY

Electrotherapy consists of the application of electrodes on the parts affected by cellulite, which stimulate the local musculature, restarting its thrust on the lymphatic vessels and thereby initiating the flow of lymph. Inexpensive, portable devices are available for sale that can be used even when watching television or reading the newspaper.

ELECTROLIPOLYSIS

Electrolipolysis (literally "electrical fat dissolution") is based on the ability of electrical current to generate pulses; introduced into the subcutis through needles, it breaks down the fat and other compounds that form the lumps.

In contrast to electrotherapy, electrolipolysis not only stimulates the muscle but also effectively destroys the cellulite tissue, thanks to the electrical impulses that can act locally with great force once the insulating barrier of the skin has been overcome.

ELECTRICAL ACUPUNCTURE

Electrical acupuncture can achieve quicker and cheaper results than electrolipolysis, which normally uses very expensive equipment. This is a technique that attempts to improve the results of traditional acupuncture (see pages 186–198).

Acupuncture needles of different lengths, depending on the thickness (up to 14 cm), when connected to the electrodes of the stimulator (equipped with a 9V battery), are inserted into the cellulite lump.

Acupuncture needles are much finer than electrolipolysis needles; for this reason, their application is extremely painless. In addition, in the case of very sensitive people, Japanese needles can be used, which are as thin as a hair and need a metal guide to prevent them from breaking.

COSMETIC SURGERY

Cosmetic surgery can be used to solve problems of severe and localized cellulite. For diffuse cellulite, though, all the methods described above can be used. However, they should be used as a first solution and even after surgery, as they improve the chances of success.

LIPOSUCTION

Liposuction, which consists of suctioning the lumpy tissue with a cannula after making several incisions in the skin, completely disrupts the delicate lymphatic circulation in a way that is practically permanent and much more so than even a well-planned and effective plastic surgery procedure. This circulatory disturbance, however, cannot guarantee that the lumps will not return within a short period of time, even if the operation went well (which is not always the case). Liposuction therefore is an extremely traumatic method, and therefore not very advisable, which can lead to serious problems such as embolisms and infections.

LYMPHATIC SELF-DRAINAGE

For minor to medium cellulite, lymphatic drainage and the recommended hygienic-dietetic, homeopathic, and phototherapeutic measures are more than enough to achieve good results. However, if you are unable to undergo regular lymphatic drainage and to engage in regular physical activity, what can you do on your own?

First, in principle, you can use electrostimulation devices, which force the muscles to do passive gymnastics. This technique is also suitable for people who are lazy or have little time.

Second, lymphatic self-drainage may be useful. Although some specialists advise against it, because all treatments should be carried out by professionals, there is no risk. If we had to call a mechanic every time a screw came loose, a bricklayer to plug a hole, or a tennis coach to play a match with friends, few people would ride a bicycle, few houses would have pictures hanging in them, and tennis clubs would be empty.

Here are the steps for some simple manipulations, in a simple and practical way.

MANIPULATIONS FOR THE FOOT, LEGS, AND BACK

FOOT MASSAGE

In medical shops and pharmacies, it is easy to find massage instruments with wheels on which the sole of the foot is vigorously rubbed by leaning on them and letting some of the weight fall off. In this way, self-massage stimulates the sole of the foot, a very important area of the body in reflexology.[9]

---

9   Reflexology, also called reflexogenic massage or zone massage, is the discipline that studies the correspondence between some parts of the body (hands and feet) and other parts of the organism.

In the foot, in fact, we find the representation of all the organs of the body; for example, in the presence of digestive discomfort caused by excess acidity in the stomach, pressure on the area of the sole corresponding to the stomach is more or less painful, depending on the severity of the organic discomfort. Similarly, massage of the area of the foot corresponding to the gastric area, if done until it no longer hurts, leads to an improvement in stomach discomfort.

Obviously, manual massage by a reflexologist is more effective than self-massage, but if it is not possible to go to the clinic every day, it is advisable to practice self-massage of the foot at least once a day, using a specific wooden tool (a tennis ball is a temporary but less effective solution).

It is best done before going to bed, preferably after a shower. To do this, rub the foot for five minutes or more; at first, you will feel many painful areas as if pricked by needles, but then the pain will be relieved and there will be a sensation of softness, sometimes associated with a slight itching. Both feet should be massaged.

The advantages of this practice are at least twofold: first, there is a generally beneficial action on the whole body and, second, there is an effective aid to lymphatic circulation, as described in the chapter on lymphatic vessels and lymph circulation mechanisms.

STROKING THE LIMBS

After massaging the foot completely, lie on your back and, while keeping one leg raised, start draining it from the back of the ankle, using both hands at the same time and without force, applying nothing more than your weight, as if caressing it.

Massage the area between the ankle and the knee five times in succession, always with the leg raised, by sliding the hands over the calves toward the back of the knee (the popliteal cavity).

The same operation is then carried out from the anterior, medial, and lateral part of the ankle to the anterior part of the knee.

Then, always with the leg raised, the inguinal pumping of the lymph is carried out, which will serve to push the lymph that has reached the inguinal lymph nodes into the pelvis toward Pecquet's cistern. The manipulation is carried out as follows: the palm of the left hand is gently placed on the groin, next to the pubis, and with the fingertips of the right hand, ten small thrusts of about 50 g are made on the left hand.

The thigh can be treated with the leg raised, as there is a kind of lymphatic ridge at the back of the thigh, approximately at the median line. For this reason, the lymph from the median area proceeds toward the groin following the inner part of the thigh, while the lymph situated laterally reaches the groin following the outer part of the thigh.

It is therefore necessary to treat first the inner part of the thigh and then the outer part, stroking each with one hand in the direction of the groin. After each phase, once drainage has been completed, groin pumping should be performed.

If, as is often the case, there are cellulite accumulations on the inside of the knee, the drainage of the inner thigh from the knee needs to be repeated more than once.

The treatment for the other leg should also be carried out step by step, following each of the instructions given.

A FEW TIPS

A good way to do this treatment is to stretch out on your back, raise your legs, and pedal for two minutes. Then bring each knee toward the chest ten times to stretch the buttocks. The tip of the right elbow should then touch the left knee with the tip of the right elbow (or as close to it as possible) and vice versa. The exercise should be repeated at least ten times.

Finally, the left leg is left hanging off the bed to stretch the buttocks and back. The exercise can be repeated by leaning on the left hip, obviously with the right leg hanging off the bed. In the morning, on waking, take a few deep breaths, bringing the arms up to activate the flow of lymph in the thoracic duct, thereby stretching the dorsal muscles and oxygenating the whole body.

During the night a cushion should always be placed under the mattress at the level of the feet to encourage the lymph to flow back from the legs to the thorax.

Chapter 9

HOW TO AVOID LEG AND CHEST DISCOMFORT

LYMPHOVENOUS INSUFFICIENCY IN THE LEGS

The formation of ectasia (dilated capillaries) on the legs or thighs, apart from the presence of cellulite, indicates venous insufficiency that is often related to lymphatic stasis. In other words, if the lymphatic system fails to sufficiently move fluids away from the legs, the venous system becomes overloaded. As a result, the more-fragile venous capillaries begin to give way. Finally, the venous walls of the larger vessels also give way, resulting in varicose veins, swollen ankles, and a feeling of widespread heaviness.

The treatment of venous insufficiency follows the same resources and remedies described for anti-cellulite treatment.

In addition, a vitamin treatment based on bioflavonoids (derived from citrus peel), vitamins A, C, and E, plus phototherapeutic substances such as Centella Asiatica (see the Phytotherapeutics in the Treatment of the Lymphatic System table on page 214), can significantly improve microcirculation.

Venoprotectant-based creams or gels can also be used.

If the person suffering from heavy legs has to stand for long hours, he or she may have to wear orthopedic stockings to prevent the veins from giving way.

A PRESCRIPTION AGAINST HEAVY LEGS

- Vitamin C extended release, 500 or 1,000 mg, one tablet per day.
- Bioflavonoids (citrus peel extracts), 500 mg, one tablet twice a day.
- Beta-carotene, one tablet twice a day.
- Wheat germ oil E200, one tablet twice a day.

The treatment lasts at least 40 days.

Sclerosing injections, which consist of the occlusion of dilated capillaries, if done properly can eliminate all or part of the unsightly capillary evidence for a certain period. However, they certainly do not improve lymphovenous circulation, but rather worsen it. Basically, it is an intervention almost always for aesthetic reasons, which is not without side effects.

Surgical intervention, involving the stripping of veins in the superficial venous circle, may be necessary when the presence of varicose veins raises fears of the development of dangerous emboli,[10] which can lead to serious pulmonary embolisms. In any case, surgical intervention must be considered as the extreme solution, so as to limit damage in an already compromised situation.

This is why the importance of prevention based on improving lymphatic circulation, through drainage, diet, physical activity, or

---

10   Embolus is a foreign element present in the blood. It can be solid, liquid, or gaseous. In the case of varicose veins, for example, it may actually be a blood clot. If an embolus obstructs a vessel, an embolism can occur.

other measures explained above, is increasingly taken into consideration.

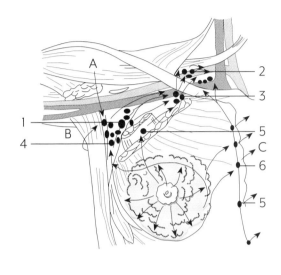

Lymphatic circulation of the breast

A. From the shoulder and back muscles

B. From the arm and back muscles

C. To contralateral lymph nodes

1. Axillary central lymph nodes

2. Supraclavicular lymph nodes

3. Subclavian lymph nodes

4. Lymph nodes under the scapulae

5. Interpectoral lymph nodes

6. Internal lymph nodes of the breast

LYMPHATIC STASIS OF THE BREAST

The breast is a glandular organ of both men and women that is poor in muscle fibers yet rich in fatty tissues. Within it, the lymphatic circulation is almost always to the axillary lymph nodes. Correct positioning of the back is therefore very important because wide intercostal breathing movements contribute to the flow of lymph in the breast tissue toward the axilla. Another lymphatic pushing mechanism is constituted by the movement of the pectoral muscles, on top of which the breast rests. All movements that favor the activity of the pectoral muscles, in particular swimming and gymnastics, contribute to lymphatic pressure and consequently to the health of the breast. Sometimes, however, excessive activity leads to bulging of the interpectoral lymph nodes, which resemble breast nodules. In this case, manual lymphatic drainage (see pages 117–118) helps to balance the lymphatic circulation and avoid tension due to lymphatic stasis.

At no time should the back be hunched and the shoulders shrugged, as the action on the spine is very detrimental.

However, the shoulders should not be carried forward either, as this reduces the range of breathing movements and increases the suspended mass. This causes lymphatic stagnation in the breast and a consequent predisposition to disease.

A very useful remedy for the prevention of lymphatic stagnation and breast nodules is a magnesium-based homeopathic product, WALA *Magnesit/Mamma comp.* The recommended dosage is between 8 and 12 granules, which should be placed directly under the tongue and allowed to melt before swallowing. They should be taken three times a day half an hour before eating. However, before starting treatment, a homeopath should be consulted.

Chapter 10

BACK PAIN AND NEURO-LYMPHATIC TREATMENT

HOW TO DETECT THE AREAS TO BE MASSAGED

In the chapter on lymph circulation (page 25), it has been pointed out that the lymph in the depression along the spine, which is formed by the relief of the back muscles, runs directly inward until it reaches the paravertebral lymph nodes and flows into the thoracic duct.

In the areas adjacent to the spine, problems related to the vertebral lymphatic circulation manifest themselves through the thickening of the connective tissue, which can be seen by massaging the patient by pinching and running the hands along the sides and over the spine, as if it were a wave. Where the pain is more acute, more attention should be paid to moving and decongesting the muscle fibers.

The disorder usually affects the damaged area, although sometimes it may be more widespread. Occasionally the lymphatic block is located on one side only, on the spine. The quickest and most effective way of working is to ask the patient where the most acute discomfort occurs.

After discovering the area to be treated, the area to be treated is pinched, in order to pinpoint the area of interest as accurately as possible and proceed with the treatment.

Apart from the area of the spine, the patient may point to another area of the back or even further away. It doesn't matter: from here a series of lines perpendicular to the spine are marked, allowing us to find those parts that need to be massaged.

Once these areas have been located, the same treatment should be continued. This manipulation is one of the simplest and most effective, which is why it is highly recommended for all those who do not have much knowledge of this discipline.

BACK MASSAGE AS A COUPLE

The exchange of a massage strengthens and restores harmony in the couple and constitutes an important and profound form of nonverbal communication as well as a message of peace.

The purpose of the massage described here, called *neuro-lymphatic treatment*, is the elimination of discomfort in the spine, almost always related to lymphatic stasis in the vertebrae, from which the pain originates.

Neuromyopathic treatment also promotes, among other things, the flow of lymph along the thoracic duct and in the paravertebral lymph nodes; it is also an important aid in preventing and counteracting cellulite, as it facilitates drainage of the areas most prone to lymphatic stagnation. Naturally, neuromyopathic treatment can also be applied to other areas of the body, making it an important, risk-free, and highly effective home remedy.

POSITION

To practice the manipulation, the patient should lie facedown on the bed. If the mattress is not sufficiently taut and hard, it is better to place some blankets on the floor and lie on them. Two cushions are needed: one under the abdomen and one under the head. The arms should be parallel to the body. The person performing the massage should sit on top of their partner's buttocks, with the knees facing outward.

If the cervical region is to be treated, the patient should sit in front of a table, on top of which there is a cushion to rest the forehead. The cervical spine should be flexed comfortably, without leaning backward. The arms should rest on the thighs.

MANIPULATION

The manipulation is more effective if, before starting, the patient takes a shower and directs a strong jet of hot water on the part to be treated.

If the pain or stiffness has been caused by cold, the affected area can be gently treated with a hot air jet from a hairdryer.

For the massage, the fingertips of the three central fingers are used, which should rest completely on the part to be treated. They are then moved in small circles; those on the right in a clockwise direction and those on the left in a counterclockwise direction. Light perpendicular pressure is applied to the most painful points. The exercise can take between 45 and 60 minutes on the right side and between 15 and 60 minutes on the left side. The pressure can vary, depending on the patient's constitution, between 20 and 100 g. For the rest of the points, it is hardly necessary to apply pressure; a light rubbing is sufficient.

At least ten rotations should be practiced for each position, always going from the highest (near the head) to the lowest. Then pinch (see pages 179–180). If the manipulation is done well, you will quickly notice that the thickness of the fold decreases and the pain diminishes, a sign that the tissues are beginning to decongest.

This massage can be done every day as often as desired until the discomfort is relieved.

In general, it is not advisable to use creams, either before or after the treatment, as this could alter the correct pressure and rubbing of the fingers (both of which are very important).

Instead, after manipulation, an arnica-based ointment can be applied, gently rubbing the area.

Some therapists will usually perform a specific acupuncture treatment for the affected area. However, given the discomfort that can occur, this should not be done more than once or twice a fortnight. If desired, it can be complemented with the massage mentioned above.

LYMPH DRAINAGE AND NATURAL MEDICINE

Chapter 11

LYMPHATIC CIRCULATION AND ACUPUNCTURE

CHINESE ACUPUNCTURE

One of the oldest therapeutic practices is Chinese acupuncture. Through continuous experimentation, the Chinese discovered the existence of a link between the health condition of the internal organs of the body and specific points on the skin surface. By puncturing certain points on the skin, they learned that a therapeutic effect is attained on certain organs.

This is possible because at the origin of diseases, there is an energy imbalance between *yin* (potential energy or matter) and *yang* (active energy or heat). If the former prevails, the latter fails and vice versa.

The energy imbalance can be general or local, but all complaints are related to each other through the meridian system (see below), a kind of fourth system (the first three are nervous, vascular, lymphatic) in which the energy flow circulates.

The skin points on which acupuncture intervenes correspond to the key points of the meridians. By acting on them, the flow of energy is modified.

VOLL'S ELECTRO-ACUPUNCTURE (EAV)

In the 1950s, the German physician Reinhold Voll (1909–1989) discovered that the acupuncture points described thousands of years earlier by Chinese physicians corresponded to small circular areas—with a higher electrical conductivity[11] concerning the surrounding skin areas—and that the electrical alteration of each point implied an alteration in the organ to which they were connected. Consequently, by measuring the electrical conductivity values of the acupuncture point or points related to a given organ, it is possible to know its possible pathological alteration. Voll also discovered that a specific therapeutic effect on an organ can be obtained not only by inserting a needle into the corresponding skin point but also by electrical stimulations applied to the same point and with a specific frequency of stimulation. This technique was called electro-acupuncture, to which the surname of its creator was added. To study the lymphatic system of each patient, specific points are used, which will be detailed in this chapter.

THE ASSESSMENT OF THE EFFECT OF PHARMACEUTICALS

Voll, after developing the electro-acupuncture technique that bears his name, discovered that contact between any substance and the skin creates a sudden electrical modification of the acupuncture points corresponding to the organ, on which the same substance has an action.

If the substance is beneficial, the points maintain or reach a normal electrical value; if it is harmful, the points show an alteration of the electrical value.

---

11   The electrical conductivity of a body means its ability to transmit electricity.

In this way, it is possible to foresee whether a certain drug will be effective or completely harmful. Voll found this out with homeopathic products, whose contact was measured electrically in each patient in order to establish the most suitable cure.

Still using this technique, in the mid-1950s, Voll foresaw, unheeded, the serious fetal disorders caused by giving a new tranquilizer, thalidomide, to pregnant women.

MERIDIANS AND THE LYMPHATIC MERIDIAN

In acupuncture, the meridian is a line, usually almost parallel to the vertical axis of the body, connecting points related to a common organ or function. By electrically measuring the points on a meridian, the state of health or disease of the corresponding organ or function can be established.

The altered values can be corrected with different methods and, at the same time, an improvement of the related organ or function can be attained. For example, a needle is inserted into the disturbed points, stimulated with electric current or massaged with local pressure (e.g., with the rounded tip of an object). In addition, a heat source can be brought near them. In fact, moxibustion is a complementary technique that consists of applying diatreme cigarettes to the point to be balanced. In other cases, a few mugwort pellets are often placed around the needle so that the needle heats up and the heat goes deeper.

In classical acupuncture, 14 main meridians are described. Two run exactly along the midline of the body, anteriorly (called Jen Mo) and posteriorly (Tou Mo). The others, in a more lateral position, run along the limbs and trunk.

Voll found eight more main meridians, among which the lymphatic meridian, at whose points the lymphatic system is represented, stands out. It starts at the thumb, runs upward along the outside of the arm, runs toward the front of the shoulder, passes over the upper margin of the trapezius near the neck, and then runs down along the cervicodorsal area toward the midline (8 cm from the sixth cervical vertebra, then 6 cm from the first thoracic vertebra, and finally 5 cm from the second thoracic vertebra). Just above the second thoracic vertebra, it joins the bladder or urogenital meridian, which runs down the back from top to bottom, almost parallel to the spine.

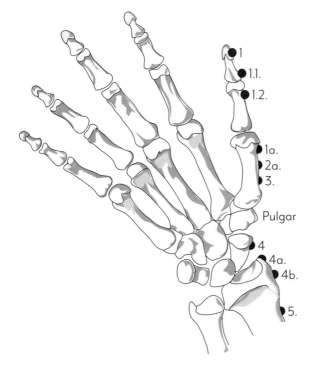

Lymph meridian points on the hand according to Voll.

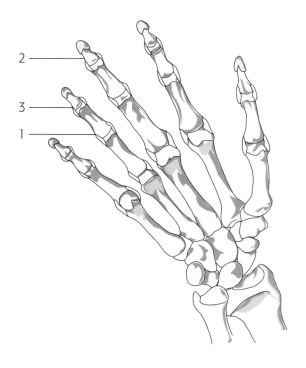

Lymphatic points of Pecquet's cistern, lymphatic vessels in the wall of arteries and veins and lymphatic stasis related to degenerative processes.

1. Pecquet's cistern point

2. Point of lymphatic vessels in the wall of arteries and veins

3. Degenerative lymphatic statis point

In total, the lymphatic meridian includes 24 points, detailed in the following table.

Correspondences Between the Acupoints and the Lymphatic System

Number from Point EAV	Position	Body or Function Related	
1	Under the lateral corner of the nail of the first toe	Palatine tonsil and peritonsillar areas	
1–1	On the lateral margin of the phalangeal margin of the first toe, before the articulation with the phalanx	Lymph flow in the ear	
1–2	On the phalanx, before the articulation with the phalanx, at the lateral border	Measures the condition of the throat lymphatic system	
1a	At the base of the phalanx of the first toe, on the lateral border	Tubal tonsil; lateral lymphatic circulation of the throat	
2	On the lateral side of the head of the first metacarpal, before the articulation with the phalanx	This point is of great importance for the assessment of dental foci (granulomas, cysts, gingival pockets, etc.), which can cause damage even in other body parts	
2a	In the middle of the first metacarpus, at the lateral edge	Lymph flow of the eye	
3	On the lateral part of the base of the first metacarpus	Lymphatic circulation of the nose and sinuses	
4	In the middle of the pulse line, at the lateral edge of the scaphoid bone	Lymph nodes and lymphatic vessels of the lung and mediastinum; bronchomediastinal trunk	

Discomfort or Characteristics	Homeopathic and Natural Remedies
This point is often activated in children	*Merc. bijod.* 5CH, three pellets every hour until improved
Hearing problems, tinnitus (ringing and buzzing), whistling, and vertigo	*Cocculus* 5CH, three pellets three times daily
Irritation and sore throat	*Merc. bijod.* 5CH, three granules six times a day; Ferr. ph. D6, three capsules a day
Otitis, ear and throat pains	Inhalations with the essence of eucalyptus
Dental pain, pyorrhea	*Merc. sol.* 5CH, three granules three times a day; Calc. fl. D6, one capsule three times a day
Any impairment of visual function; conjunctivitis, blepharitis	Eye drops based on eyebright; *Pulsatilla* 5CH, three granules three times a day
Cold, chronic rhinitis, sinusitis	*Luffa* 5CH in aerosol in case of allergy; *Stannum* 5CH, three granules three times a day in case of chronic complaints
Tracheitis, tracheobronchitis, bronchitis, pneumonia	*Ant. tart.* 4CH, three granules six times a day

Correspondences Between the Acupoints and the Lymphatic System

Number from Point EAV	Position	Body or Function Related	
4a	The apex of the stylohyoid process of the radius, near the pulse line	Lymph from the esophagus	
4b	At about 5 mm above 4a	Lymphatic circulation of throat and pharynx	
5	On the lateral side of the radius, in the hollow formed by the bone at its base, 1 cm above point 4b	Lymphatic circulation of the heart	
6	At the lateral edge of the radius, 4 to 5 cm above point 5	Lymphatic circulation of the arm and breast region	
7	On the lateral margin of the radius, between the brachioradialis muscle and the extensor carpi longus, 4 cm from the elbow crease	Intestinal lymphatic trunk and mesenteric lymph nodes	
7a	2 cm above point 7	Lymph flow from the digestive organs, sometimes flowing in a single celiac duct, itself a tributary of the intestinal duct	
8	At the radial terminal part of the elbow crease	Lymph nodes mesoscopic and rectosigmoid lymph nodes; colonic lymph flow; lymph nodes of the elbow	

Discomfort or Characteristics	Homeopathic and Natural Remedies
Hiatal hernia, gastroesophageal reflux	*Kal. carb.* 4CH, three granules four times daily
—	*Phytolacca* 5CH, three granules three times a day
Palpitations, bronchial sounds, precordial pains	*Arnica* 5CH, three granules three times daily
Arm pain and discomfort, asthma	*Symphitum* 4CH, three granules three times a day. Asthma: *Ipeca* 4CH and *Arum triph.* 4CH, three pellets of each, alternated until improvement
Intestinal discomfort of any kind	Intestinal ferments
Digestion discomfort	*Argentum nitricum* 5CH, three granules three times daily
Colitis, constipation, epicondylitis	Colitis and constipation: *Podophyllum* 5CH, three pellets three times daily; epicondylitis: *Ruta* 5CH, three pellets three times daily

Correspondences Between the Acupoints and the Lymphatic System

Number from Point EAV	Position	Body or Function Related	
9	4 cm above point 8, between the biceps and the brachioradialis muscle	Lymphatic circulation of endocrine and breast lymph nodes	
9a	On the lateral margin of the humerus, next to the lower apex of the deltoid muscle	Periaortic lymphatic plexus and aortic lymph nodes	
10	At the upper extremity of the bicipital hollow of the humerus, on the humeral insertion of the pectoralis major	Lumbar lymph nodes and lymphatic vessels	
10a	On the lower margin of the clavicle in the space between the deltoid and the pectoralis, on the medial margin of the deltoid	Axillary lymph nodes and lymph flow; subclavian lymphatic trunk	
10b	At the lower margin of the clavicle, in the space between the deltoid and the pectoralis, at the margin of the latter	On the left, the cervical part of the thoracic duct and, on the right, the large right lymphatic vein	

Discomfort or Characteristics	Homeopathic and Natural Remedies
Endocrine disruption	*Pituitary and hypothalamus* 7CH, three pellets of each type on alternate nights
Abdominal discomfort, colic	*Magn. ph. D6,* one capsule every hour until improved
Back pain, lumbago, colitis, constipation, chronic urogenital inflammations, menstrual pains, etc.	*Rhus tox* 5CH, three pellets three times daily
Trauma and muscle sprains and strains of the shoulder and pectoral muscles, mastopathies (diseases of the breast)	—
Inflammatory complaints or trauma of the neck and arm, sometimes at the same time as complaints of the organs of the chest and abdomen	—

Correspondences Between the Acupoints and the Lymphatic System

Number from Point EAV	Position	Body or Function Related	
11	2.5 cm above the clavicle, in the intramuscular space called the infraclavicular fossa. 1.5 cm below the apex of the fossa, at the lower margin of the scalene muscle and the lateral margin of the sternocleidomastoid muscle	It flows into the subclavian vein from the main lymphatic ducts	
12	1.5 cm above and behind point 11, at the front edge of the trapezium	Lymph nodes of the stomach	
13	At the posterior margin of the upper line of the trapezius, 5 cm from the posterior part of the sixth cervical vertebrae	Lymphatic circulation of the bile ducts and gallbladder	
14	At the level of the posterior part of the first dorsal vertebra and 3 cm from the midline	Lymph nodes and lymphatic circulation of the urogenital organs and pelvis	

In addition to the lymph points located on the lymphatic meridian, there are other acupuncture points located on other meridians and corresponding to other sectors of the lymphatic system. On this and the following pages, the most important ones are identified.

Discomfort or Characteristics	Homeopathic and Natural Remedies
General "thermometer" or "lymphometer" of the state of the entire lymphatic system	*Castanea vesca* D1 and *Sorbus domestica* D1 (gemmotherapy), 30 drops of each in a little water three times a day before meals
Gastritis	*Ficus carica* D1 (gemmotherapy), 50 drops in a little water, three times daily before meals
Abdominal bloating after dinner, pain or discomfort in the right hypochondrium, bilateral cramps	*Chelidonium* 5CH, three granules three times daily
Urogenital infections, pelvic trauma, hemorrhoids	—

Other Points Corresponding to the Lymphatic System

Name and Point EAV Point Number	Position	
Meridian point of circulation (8a)	On the palm of the hand, on the lateral margin of the third metacarpal, below the metacarpophalangeal joint	
Meridian point of the "triple heater" (16a)	1.5 cm below the mastoids, in the middle of the sternocleidomastoid muscle	
Circulation meridian (8b)	On the lateral margin of the third toe, near the metatarsophalangeal joint	
Circulation meridian (8f)	On the lateral margin of the phalanx of the third toe, close to the articulation with the phalange	
Bazopancreatic meridian (9)	In the depression of the inferior border of the medial condyle of the tibia, at the level of the apex	

Body or Function Related	Discomfort or Characteristics	Remedios Homeopathic and Natural
The thoracic duct on the left; lymphatic granvena on the right or right chest wall lymphatic circulation	Lymphatic system warning point	—
Deep cervical lymph nodes; lower cervical lymph nodes; lower auricular lymph nodes	Sore throats, neck pains, stiff neck, tooth and gum problems	—
Pecquet's cistern	Warning on the lymphatic circulation of all abdominal organs	—
Lymphatic circulation of the lymphatic vessel wall (vasa lymphatica vasorum)	Circulatory problems (arteriosclerosis, Buerger's disease, Raynaud's disease, diabetes, metabolic disorders, hypertension)	*Olea europaea* D1 (gemmotherapy) and *Cercis sil.* D1, 30 drops of each in a little water before three daily meals
Lymphatic circulation of the legs and knees	Venous and lymphatic insufficiency, edema of the ankles, abdominal swelling, enuresis (loss of urine during the night), menstrual irregularities, osteoarthritis and trauma to the knee, especially to the meniscus	For lymphovenous insufficiency: bioflavonoids, *Aesculus hippocastanum*, *Hamamelis*, Centella asiatica, vitamin A, and vitamin E. Centella can be taken externally

Chapter 12

LYMPHATIC CIRCULATION AND HOMEOPATHY

HISTORY AND PRINCIPLES OF HOMEOPATHY

Homeopathy, derived from the Greek words *ómoios* ("similar") and *pathos* ("sensitivity" or "disease"), was conceived of by the German physician Samuel Hahnemann (1755–1843).

Hahnemann observed that workers who worked with quinine, used in malaria cures, often had symptoms similar to those of malaria (periodic fevers), although in fact they were caused by malaria poisoning.

By contrast, mercury, which was used in the treatment of syphilis, and which is characterized by the formation of ulcers on the mucous membranes, could cause the same conditions in cases of overdose.

Arsenic, used in small quantities as both a tonic and a remedy for anemia and colitis, if administered in excess, produced anemia and colitis that could be fatal.

Appreciating these observations, Hahnemann diluted some substances (which were toxic if given in large doses) and experimented with their effects. Subsequently, he observed that the effects were more potent if they were shaken vertically when diluted. This procedure was called dynamization or potentization.

Disregarding medical nosology, Hahnemann analyzed the symptoms of each patient. At the same time, he began to experiment on himself and other healthy people with the effect of various diluted and dynamized substances. Each substance produced specific symptoms in the healthy individual.

Hahnemann then compared the symptoms produced in healthy people with those of the individual patient and prescribed to each patient the substance that produced a series of symptoms in the healthy person similar to those of the sick person. The German physician thereby discovered the therapeutic effects of dynamized substances.

How is it possible, though, that homeopathic substances, so diluted (down to one part per million), produce therapeutic effects? A decisive proof in favor of Hahnemann came in the 1950s from Voll, who discovered a method for assessing the effect of medicines (see page 186). According to him, these would act through the radiant effect obtained in their preparation, starting from a base substance, then progressively diluted and dynamized in a vertical direction.

In fact, research carried out in the 1950s and 1960s at the University of Milan and the 1970s and 1980s at the University of Vienna demonstrated that the cells of the body "communicate" with each other through radiation produced by the DNA of the cell nucleus, which emits and receives intercellular signals, allowing the organization of the collective activity of the different cell groups.

According to the same research, the disease is caused by a dysfunction in the exchange of radiant information between cell and cell, resulting in a disturbance of the electrical potential of the cell membrane. From a clinical point of view, it manifests itself in the form of functional symptoms (such as intermittent or periodic pain, discomfort, or ill-defined discomfort) which lead to a chemical alteration (detected by blood tests) and, finally, reveal structural deformations that can be detected by radiological tests or ultrasound scans.

HELPING YOURSELF AND OTHERS

In the following pages, the reader will find some homeopathic remedies that can be very effective in the treatment of complaints that are often related to lymphatic stasis of certain lymphonodal stations. These remedies can be used alone or in conjunction with lymphatic massage.

THE DISCOVERY OF RADIATION FROM MEDICINES

One day, Voll, during an electro-acupuncture seminar, measured the prostatic point (located on the foot) of an assistant suffering from prostatic hypertrophy, whose most common symptom was difficulty urinating.

The point value was altered and had a lower electrical conductivity than normal. Voll then measured the prostate point of the other attendees and, to verify this, also the point of the first attendee, who in the meantime had put on his jacket because he was cold. Surprisingly, Voll saw that the point value had normalized.

Since the only different element was the jacket (which was missing in the first measurement), the assistant was asked to remove it, and the prostate point was measured again. Again it was altered. The assistant put the jacket back on and his prostate point returned to the normal electrical conductivity value.

What was in the American? Perhaps the solution to cure prostatic hypertrophy.

The assistant took off his jacket but took the medicine in his hand: the point value was normal, altering again when the assistant put down the medicine.

Voll concluded that the body is sensitive to radiation coming from any substance, specific to its chemical constitution. When the body detects, even through the skin, a signal coming from a substance that has a therapeutic effect, the electrical values of the acupuncture points, if altered, return to normal.

By contrast, if toxic radiation affects the skin, the acupuncture points show a pathological electrical disturbance.

It should be noted, however, that each lymphatic stasis has a precise cause that must be understood. For example, a dental focus (inflammation of a tooth) causes lymphatic stasis in the submaxillary area, which is why it is necessary to see a dentist.

HOMOTOXICOLOGY

This is a medical discipline that developed in the 1950s thanks to the research of H. H. Reckeweg on the application of biochemical and toxicological principles to homeopathy. According to Reckeweg, the reason why the body becomes ill lies in the fact that certain metabolic stages are, in some cases, blocked by toxins that can be bacterial, fungal, viral, chemical, chemical-physical, or just physical (such as certain types of radiation).

Bioelectronic methods are used for diagnosis, especially Voll's electro-acupuncture (see page 186), which can detect the exact type of toxin. In addition, a good anamnesis and an objective examination of the patient can help diagnose the symptoms and signs produced by the toxin.

The therapy consists of removing the toxin from the biochemical compound (enzyme, protein, coenzyme, cell membrane components, mitochondria, etc.) to which it binds and thereby blocks its action.

Reckeweg used the same toxins diluted homeopathically. For example, in the case of a throat condition caused by hemolytic streptococcus, he administered this toxin suitably diluted so that its elimination was stimulated.

In addition to taking advantage of the depurative action and the ability to bind toxins and carry them out of the organism that these so-called homotoxicological remedies possessed (whose application resembles that of the homeopathic micro vaccines developed by the German physician Hering in the last century), Reckeweg used homeopathically prepared physiological metabolites of the Krebs cycle[12] capable of activating the interrupted metabolic stage by supplying them after the hemotoxin (i.e., the homeopathic toxin), which made it possible to remove the real toxin from the organism. On the one hand, the organism was purified and, on the other hand, functional restructuring and regeneration of the injured tissues was undertaken.

However, the *grundsystem* (pages 17–24), conceived as the anatomical and functional site where diseases manifest themselves or not, and against which battles are won or lost, can't be forgotten. Indeed, this conception is reminiscent of the concepts of Rudolf Virchow, a famous Berlin anatomopathologist of the last century, according to whom every disease is caused by an alteration of the cell. With Reckeweg, the vision of the *grundsystem* as the basic frontier of health represents both an evolution and a complement to Virchow's concepts.

---

12   This is the most important metabolic cycle, during which the different biochemical steps occur that allow the body to extract energy from food and synthesize its constituents, such as muscle proteins.

In any case, the homeopathic remedy corresponding to the stasis and the symptoms present can be used both to prevent their worsening and to achieve a faster and more complete healing after dental treatment.

SCHÜSSLER SALTS

Schüssler's salts are homeopathic remedies prepared by the German physician Wilhelm Schüssler (1821–1898). They are twelve in number and represent the salts that are always found in human ashes after cremation.

Schüssler believed that a deficiency of each of these salts could induce specific symptoms and that, in order to avoid this deficiency, the best remedy was to supply either the missing salt or salts homeopathically.

The most common form in which Schüssler's salts are used is D6, i.e., dilution and dynamization, which takes place in six successive stages, in each of which the salt is diluted ten times. Schüssler's salts are available in tablet form, to be dissolved under the tongue three times a day, at least 30 minutes before eating; they are also available in an ointment form, with the same dynamization, and should be applied where necessary: eczema, burns, blemishes, scars, and so on. For a more potent effect, they can be administered in tablet and ointment form at the same time.

The salts, in addition to being used for each specific symptom, are also helpful as remedies for the lymphatic system, in the case of impaired lymphatic circulation in the different parts of the body.

Schüssler Salts, Symptoms, and Healed Lymphatic Areas

Salt	Main Symptoms	Lymphatic Area
Kalium phosporicum (potassium phosphate, KH_2PO_4)	Anxiety, tiredness, lack of energy, teething problems (with *Calcium fluoratum*)	Head
Natrum sulfuricum (sodium sulphate, Na_2SO_4)	Moodiness, melancholy, digestive discomfort with a feeling of discomfort in the liver; discomfort in the left lung	Neck. It usually acts in the key lymph nodes—confluence of the lymph of the neck and arm and in the terminal part of the thoracic duct and the left broncho-diastinal duct
Kalium chloratum or muriaticum (potassium chloride, KCl)	Disorders of the respiratory tract, from the ear downward: otitis media, eustachian tube catarrh, thrush, pharyngitis, bronchitis, pneumonia with dense and viscous white and grayish exudations due to the presence of fibrin; eye complaints: conjunctivitis, chorioretinitis; breast complaints: mastitis; pre-patellar bursitis due to exertion and in growing children	Lymph from thoracic organs and bronchomediastinal trunks; used in the healing of pleuritis with exudations to prevent the formation of adhesions
Calcium fluoratum (calcium fluoride, CaF_2)	Difficult dentition, discomfort of tendons, ligaments, cartilage, bones, periosteum, paradental tissue (pyorrhea), venous wall	Lymphatic circulation of the cervical spine, back, and thorax; thoracic route of the lymphatic duct, dorsal paravertebral lymph nodes, intercostal and parasternal lymphatics

Schüssler Salts, Symptoms, and
Healed Lymphatic Areas

Salt	Main Symptoms	Lymphatic Area
Magnesium phosphoricum (magnesium phosphate, $MgHPO_4 + 3H_2O$)	Spasms and colic, cramps, severe coughing, nerve conduction disturbances in the heart	Lymphatic circulation of the heart
Kalium sulfuricum (potassium sulphide, K_2SO_4)	Depression, tearfulness; thick yellow mucus, digestive, and genital mucous membranes; intermittent rheumatic pains; popular skin eruptions; lymphatic stasis in legs	Pecquet's cistern, the point of confluence of lymph from the abdominal organs and the legs
Natrium phosphoricum (sodium monohydrogen phosphate, $Na KPO_{24} + 12H_2O$)	Heartburn, hyperacidity, diarrhea related to digestive discomfort with a feeling of heartburn and hyperacidity	Lymph from the gastrointestinal and intestinal lymphatic ducts
Calcium sulfuricum (precipitated calcium sulphate, $CaS_4 + 2H_2O$)	Suppurative processes of all kinds, venereal infections, phlegmons	Lymphatic circulation of genital organs and lymph nodes inguinal

Schüssler Salts, Symptoms, and Healed Lymphatic Areas

Salt	Main Symptoms	Lymphatic Area
Silica (silicic acid, $SiO_2 + 2H_2O$)	Dystrophy, rickets, skin irregularities, fistulas, tubercular processes of various organs, growth disturbances of skin adnexa: striated hair and nails; sores between the toes, allergic respiratory tract complaints and skin eczema, abdominal swelling together with weakness, particularly in the extremities	Lymphatic circulation of the arm, subclavian duct, and lymphatic circulation of the thigh
Calcium phosphoricum (calcium phosphate, $CaHPO_4 + 2H_2O$)	Lack of physical and mental dynamism, skin irregularities in children, night sweats, especially in children, delayed teething, delayed closure of the fontanels	Popliteal lymph nodes, knee discomfort; in children, lymphonodal swellings in the auricular lymph nodes
Natrium chloratum or muriaticum (sodium chloride, $NaCl$)	Loss of appetite, asthenia, anemia, chronic catarrh of the back of the mouth, gingivitis	Lymphatic circulation of the ankle and the front of the neck, especially the larynx and thyroid
Ferrum phosphoricum (iron phosphate, $FePO_4 + 4H_2O$)	Fever, sore and red throat, neck pain caused by muscle tension, thyroiditis and otitis, tiredness or stiffness of the foot muscles with metatarsalgia due to postural alteration	Lymphatic circulation of the large superficial muscles of the neck and feet

Chapter 13

LYMPH AND PHYTOTHERAPY

Phytotherapy includes all natural remedies that use substances of plant origin, i.e., plants or parts of plants (roots, flowers, leaves, fruits, and so on), or substances derived from their infusion, distillation, and the like. When used to stimulate proper lymph circulation, numerous plant-derived medicines do *not* produce side effects.

GEMMOTHERAPY

The gemmotherapy products come from the treatment of plant bud substances, diluted tenfold in relation to the original mother substance (and indicated by the acronym D1), which places them very close to homeopathic products, often used by French homeopaths.

They are usually marketed in 30 or 50 ml bottles.

The average dose is usually 30 drops, administered three times a day before each meal and diluted in a little mineral water. The duration of the cure is about 40 days. The remedies can be taken together, although it is not advisable to take more than 60 drops per dose.

Gemmotherapeutics in the Treatment of the Lymphatic System

Gemmotherapy Remedy Aches	Pains Cured
Aesculus hippocastanum D1	Lymphovenous insufficiency, cellulitis, hemorrhoids, cold with nasal congestion
Castanea vesca D1	Lymphovenous insufficiency, cellulitis, hemorrhoids, heavy legs, varicose veins
Ribes nigrum D1	Hemorrhoids (with Aesculus hippocastanum), varicose veins (with Sorbus domestica); anti-inflammatory action
Rosa canina D1	Vascular fragility; thanks to its vitamin C content, it strengthens the vein walls
Sorbus domestica D1	Same indications as for Castanea vesca, with which it is almost always associated in therapy
Vitis vinifera D1	Tired legs, heavy legs, varicose veins, hemorrhoids, dilated capillaries, and reddening of the face; also available in tablet decongestant and astringent action; stimulates the immune activity of lymphocytes
Zea mays D1	Cellulite; diuretic action (to be combined with other therapies)

The main remedies useful for normalizing lymphatic circulation are described below. Obviously, the results will be much better if the remedies are combined with lymphatic drainage techniques carried out by a specialist (pages 72–153) or by oneself (pages 170–173).

A GEMMOTHERAPY RECIPE AGAINST CELLULITE

The first phase of treatment:

- Sorbus domestica D1 (chemotherapy);
- Castanea vesca D1 (chemotherapeutic);
- Aesculus hippocastanum D1 (chemotherapeutic).

Before three meals, drink 20 drops of each type diluted in a little still water. The treatment should continue until the bottles are used up.

The second phase of treatment:

- Betula pubescens D1 (chemotherapy);
- Quercus pedunculata D1 (chemotherapeutic).

Before three meals, drink 20 drops of each type diluted in a little water. The treatment should be continued until the bottles are used up.

Start the cycle again from the first phase (Sorbus, Castanea, and Aesculus), continue with the second phase and start again, bearing in mind that the duration of treatment is at least 40 days. However, it is advisable to consult a specialist before starting treatment.

PHYTOTHERAPY

Phytotherapeutic products in tablet form are normally packaged separately. In addition, the preparation of the tablets reduces the active ingredients.

It is sufficient to take one tablet three times a day before each meal. The treatment usually lasts 40 days and can be combined with other phytotherapeutic products.

EXTERNAL-USE CREAMS AGAINST CELLULITE

Various natural creams are available for sale, all of which a pharmacist, herbalist, or lymphatic drainage specialist can recommend. Some of them have a certain action on the local metabolism, so they should be applied after massaging the skin with a brush or a thick sponge so that the superficial circulation is activated and will lead to better absorption of the cream's ingredients.

If you do not want to use industrially produced creams, you can prepare the following:

- 100 g moisturizing cream
- 1 drop of essence of each of the following plants: Aesculus, Arnica, Hamamelis, Hydrastis, Peony, Pulsatilla, and Ruscus.

VITAMIN INTEGRATORS

Vitamin integrators for microcirculation and tone of venous and lymphatic vessels are as follows:

- Vitamin A (cranberry, black currant, and carrot extract);
- Vitamin E (wheat germ oil);
- Vitamin C (citrus fruits);
- bioflavonoids (citrus peel).

Phytotherapeutics in the Treatment of the Lymphatic System

Phytotherapeutics	Disorders
Birch	Fluid retention due to thyroid insufficiency; carries minerals and stimulates thyroid activity
Chicory	Vascular fragility: protects microcirculation and strengthens the venous wall
Artichoke	Venous and lymphatic insufficiency; cellulitis with abdominal swelling (after eating)

Phytotherapeutics in the Treatment of the Lymphatic System

Phytotherapeutics	Disorders
Alfalfa	Stimulates white blood cell and lymphocyte activity; indicated for anemia and influenza
Seaweed	Discomfort cured or in the process of disappearing
Boldo	Venous and lymphatic insufficiency, cellulite; diuretic action
Milk thistle	Similar use to boldo; can be used together
Asian pennywort	Action similar to boldo and artichoke; can be taken together or alternately
Cumin	Diabetic vascular insufficiency; stimulates enzymatic and endocrine activity of the pancreas
Damiana	Venous insufficiency with digestive difficulties (gastric origin)
Echinacea	Cellulite (in stressed women); tonic and aphrodisiac action
Equisetum	Osteoporosis, rickets; diuretic and calcifying action
Escholtzia	Lymphatic stasis, frequent infectious diseases with loss of appetite; stimulates the immune system
Eucalyptus	Lymphatic stasis, depression of the immune system in asthenic and insomnia sufferers
Fenugreek	Immune insufficiency, frequent respiratory discomfort
Glucomannan	Supports proper lymphatic flow in the breast; especially in lactation, is a general tonic; promotes milk let-down and maintains lactation
Black and red currants	Protective of microcirculation; strengthens the lymphatic and venous vessel wall

Phytotherapeutics in the Treatment of the Lymphatic System

Phytotherapeutics	Disorders
Ispaghol	Venous insufficiency and cellulitis associated with constipation; facilitates the formation and expulsion of feces; indications similar to glucomannan
Melissa	Lymphatic stasis associated with intestinal and menstrual pain, anxiety; soothing and antispasmodic action
Nettle	Diuretic and mineralizing action
Orthosiphon	Purifying, diuretic and slimming action; very useful in slimming diets
Papaya	Digestive difficulties, especially with grains; digestive and diuretic action
Thinking	Lymphatic stasis in the head, associated with acne and skin irregularities
Pilosella	Cellulite, edema; useful in slimming diets
Grapefruit	Cellulite; useful in slimming diets
Rhubarb	Constipation with abdominal bloating, and lymphovenous insufficiency; stimulates biliary activity
Taraxacum	Diuretic; also regulates bile flow, digestion, and intestinal transit; useful against cellulite and lymphatic stasis in general

VEGETABLE JUICES AND WFPS

Plant juices have a higher amount of active ingredients than tablets, but they have to be stored in the refrigerator and are also more expensive. WFPS (whole solutions of fresh plants, micronized, frozen, and preserved in alcohol) are an intermediate solution between juices and tablets: they can even be kept outside the refrigerator, and the only drawback is if they have to be carried around, as the 100 cc containers are quite heavy and take up a certain amount of space.

SEAWEED

Seaweed baths are very effective in the treatment of cellulite, as a bath rich in salts contained in seaweed is equivalent to osmotic drainage.[13] In addition, the iodine in seaweed stimulates local metabolism and promotes the exchange of nutrients and waste between cells.

DIURETIC AND ANTI-CELLULITE THERAPY BASED ON VEGETABLE JUICES

- First week: nettle and hock leaf
- Second week: dandelion and horsetails
- Third week: celery and watercress
- Fourth week: artichoke and watercress

One tablespoon of each juice should be diluted in 12 tablespoons of water, and taken before the three main meals. The treatment should last about eight weeks. In addition, at least one liter of mineral water should be drunk between meals.

---

13   On the osmotic process, see page 10.

Chapter 14

LYMPH AND BACH FLOWERS

BACH FLOWER THERAPY

Edward Bach (1886–1936) graduated in medicine in 1912 from the University of Birmingham, England, and worked as a microbiologist at University College Hospital in London until 1918, when he moved to the London Homeopathic Hospital. He perfected seven types of vaccines to combat some chronic diseases; he then prepared the same vaccines through a homeopathic procedure to maintain efficacy and eliminate unpleasant effects. He concluded that a correct diet is basic for the prevention and cure of diseases.

At the same time, Bach observed the important role played by negative emotions in the onset and development of illnesses. In order to cure the psychological complaints of his patients, he studied the therapeutic effect of 37 common flowers. He then added the 38th remedy: mineral water (rock water).

But what are the principles and the cases on which Bach flower therapy is based?

THE EFFECTS OF THE PSYCHE ON DISEASE AND VICE VERSA

As has been known for thousands of years by traditional medicine and in particular in Chinese medicine, every psychic or emotional state is related to an organ or an organic function.

For example, the liver and bile ducts become diseased due to the persistence of emotions of anger or antagonism. By contrast, a hepatobiliary disorder (e.g. viral hepatitis) produces angry reactions in the patient.

Unexpected grief (loss, disappointment, bereavement, and so forth) causes cardiac discomfort; in turn, heart disease reduces happiness of life and enthusiasm.

Worries, persistent thoughts, and difficult decisions cause stomach discomfort; in turn, a chronic stomach sufferer develops an overly worried or pensive character. Anxiety causes lung discomfort, and respiratory diseases cause anxiety.

A sudden fright, too much effort, or too great a responsibility causes discomfort in the kidneys and urinary tract. Similarly, a kidney patient suffers from character disorders related to fear (phobias), willpower (abulia or stubbornness), and responsibility (tendency to take it all on or leave it all behind).

LYMPHATIC STASIS AND EMOTIONS

Lymphatic stasis in the microcirculation (see the chapter on *grundsystem,* page 17) is one of the first phenomena in the pathological chain, which becomes increasingly evident even on clinical examination, with signs such as swelling and muscle contractures.

PREPARATION, MECHANISM OF ACTION, AND POSOLOGY

The flower is placed in spring water for several hours and exposed to light; the therapeutic essence of the flower is transferred to the water, or rather, the sunlight is transferred to the water.

The liquid obtained, when suitably diluted and dynamized (see page 201), is given to the patient; alcohol is used to preserve the remedy.

Today, Bach flowers are sold in pharmacies and herbalists' shops in concentrated bottles. Their contents must be diluted and energized before use.

Although the preparation technique of the flower remedy is different from the homeopathic remedy, the effect of Bach flowers is not chemical, but rather "vibrational," i.e., physical: the flower leaves its electromagnetic trace in the water, which picks up the therapeutic effect, as happens in the case of homeopathic medicines.

Precisely for this reason, what we have said about Voll's method of measuring the efficacy of medicines (see page 186), can also be verified in the therapeutic effect of Bach flowers. In fact, if the flower remedy that cures the negative emotion which is the cause of the physical discomfort is brought into contact with the body of a sick person, an instantaneous improvement is noticed in the electrical values of the acupuncture points corresponding to the diseased organ(s).

In the treatment of lymphatic stasis, it is advisable to administer only the chosen flower remedy, and not together with other flower remedies, in the evening, before going to bed. The dose is five drops directly under the tongue or diluted in a little mineral water. Do not swallow for two minutes.

Delivery, repeated even three or four times during the day, loses effectiveness and can provoke unpleasant emotions.

A negative emotion acts on the microcirculation, increasing the flow of plasma between cells and preventing its normal outflow. This leads to tissue swelling and consequently to lymphatic stasis, which in turn prevents the correct nutritional supply to the cell and the removal of waste products.

The lack of proper nutrition and the progressive accumulation of waste products give rise to diseases. If lymphatic stasis is long-lasting, the disease can become more and more serious.

Lymphatic drainage allows the correct circulation of the lymph to be reestablished, solving any stasis problems that may arise. However, if the emotional cause is not resolved, the problem is likely to recur. Here lies the importance of flower remedies, which can solve the source of lymphatic stasis of the microcirculation.

BACH FLOWERS AND LYMPHATIC STASIS

As mentioned above, each flower can act on a specific emotional discomfort, which in turn can produce lymphatic stasis in the organ affected by that type of emotion.

Bach divided the 38 remedies he discovered into seven categories, each of which represents a type of emotion that tends to alter one or more organic functions. These categories are as follows:
- abashment and despair;
- disinterest in the present;
- excessive concern;
- hypersensitivity;
- insecurity;
- fear;
- loneliness.

In the following, only remedies useful for solving problems related to lymphatic stasis will be considered.

DEJECTION AND DESPAIR

The remedies in this category act on psychosomatic problems of the lungs, with catarrh and lymphatic stasis in the thorax.

LARCH

This flower remedy is indicated for those who are depressed by a constant sense of inferiority. It should also be remembered that larch resin resolves lymphatic stasis of the chest and respiratory tract catarrh.

DISINTEREST IN THE PRESENT

People feel an alienation from reality, a difficult tolerance of life and repeated mistakes. The most affected part is the circulatory system.

WHITE CHESTNUT

The flower of the Indian chestnut has a positive effect on disturbing thoughts and on the worries that are constantly present in the head, taking away peace and making life heavy. It promotes lymphovenous circulation in the legs, when these extremities swell and weigh almost like thoughts.

WILD ROSE

Rosehip acts on the lymphatic circulation and the lymph nodes of the throat; it relieves the feeling of sluggishness and the inability to overcome a period of difficulty, particularly heavy. The fruit of the same plant, which is rich in vitamin C, is very useful in the prevention and treatment of flu and cold complaints.

EXCESSIVE CONCERN

This category includes remedies suitable for people who show excessive care for others, who are overly concerned about what others think of them, or who suffer from an inferiority complex because they have not done their best for someone.

Such remedies act in a beneficial way on the brain, nervous system, blood pressure, digestion, and lymphatic stasis of the neck and face.

VINE

This flower is very effective in relieving both excessive focus on others, which can lead to inferiority complexes, and lymphatic stasis discomfort related to this state of mind.

HYPERSENSITIVITY

Hypersensitive people often suffer physically from muscle and joint problems.

CENTAURY

The feeling relieved by this flower remedy is physical and mental exhaustion resulting from excessive activity (of joint mobility) performed to help others, due to an excess of altruism or expenditure of one's own energies.

INSECURITY

The main object of the remedies of the second category is the stomach. Here we will talk in particular about gentian.

GENTIAN

We know from herbal medicine that gentian root has a digestive action. Gentian flower relieves feelings of indecision and soothes the digestive system. In fact, insecurity causes functional digestive insufficiency and abdominal lymphatic stasis, with gas formation in the intestine, belching, and flatulence.

FEAR

The first category, which obviously also includes the different types of anxiety, comprises five remedies:

- Aspen;
- Cherry plum;
- Mimulus;
- Red chestnut;
- Rock rose.

These flowers have a healing action on the kidneys, urinary tract, lungs, respiratory tract, and vascular system of the head, eyes, and ears, but also on the stomach (fear and worry together) and the uterus or prostate (fear for relatives).

ASPEN

It is effective in cases of respiratory problems, including allergies. The main feeling is disturbance at any event, even minor ones.

CHERRY PLUM

It is a remedy for stomach discomfort associated with swelling of the ankle (lymphatic stasis of the legs) or of the limbs, which are always cold. The feelings associated with this discomfort are the fear of not doing something right or of producing unwanted effects.

MIMULUS

It cures lymphatic stasis of the eye, which can lead to impaired visual function, as well as all problems in the orbital region (bags under the eyes). The most frequently related feelings are fear of the dark and fear of daily chores.

RED CHESTNUT

It resolves problems of localized lymphatic stasis in the uterus and prostate. The related feeling is the constant fear that someone close to you will suffer an unforeseen mishap.

ROCK ROSE

It is recommended for lymphatic stasis due to physical and mental disorders, especially in the head, such as reduced or impaired hearing, tinnitus (ringing and whistling in the ears), vertigo, and loss of balance. The corresponding feelings are dizziness and alienation.

SOLEDAD

The feeling of loneliness can affect even people who appear to be perfectly integrated into social life. Moreover, loneliness-related depression is known to be one of the great evils of the modern age.

HEATHER

Heather lightens the feelings of those who on the one hand want to be alone and, on the other hand, want company. Its psychosomatic action influences the kidneys, the skin, and the lungs, which are purifying organs designed to remove waste from the body (i.e., to leave the body alone, unaccompanied by waste). If the cleansing action of the kidneys and lungs is lacking, toxins concentrate in the lymphatic vessels of the dermis (the deepest part of the skin) of the face, shoulders, hands, and feet and can then lead to eczema and acne.

Chapter 15

LYMPHATIC CIRCULATION REPRESENTED IN THE IRIS

BRIEF PRESENTATION OF IRIDOLOGY

Iridology is a very ancient medical specialty that has been developed in both the West and the East. It consists of the study of the iris (the colored part of the eye), in the center of which is the pupil, which regulates the flow of light to the retina.

The study of the iris is particularly useful in determining the state of health of all the organs of the body. In fact, the parts into which the iris can be divided, according to the indications of a map that has been drawn up over hundreds of years of observation, correspond specifically to certain organs or functions of the body, in a similar way to acupuncture points. According to this medical trend, the state of nourishment and well-being of each organ or function is picked up by the nervous system and transferred to the iris, just as if it were the monitor on a computer.

In fact, the iris is the only part of the body where the state of health of the organs can be seen directly. If an organ suffers and its nutritional status is poor, the corresponding part of the iris shows a lack of nourishment. A darker color may appear, due to the thinning of the superficial layers of the iris, or a lighter color, which reveals the black back part (which corresponds to the front part of the retina). Pigments sometimes appear at the same time, corresponding to the deposit of waste, due to the malfunctioning of purification, particularly lymphatic purification.

IRIS STRUCTURE

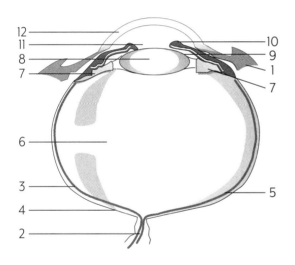

Diagram of the eye in cross-section.

1. Conjunctiva
2. Optic nerve
3. Retina
4. Choroids
5. Sclerotic
6. Vitreous body
7. Ciliary bodies
8. Crystalline lens
9. Rear camera
10. Iris
11. Anterior chamber
12. Cornea

The iris is shaped like a coin with a hole in the center. Its innermost part is a sort of extension of the retina, which in the anterior part of the eye has no sensory function and is something like the diaphragm of a camera. It is made up of different layers of cells and gradually increases in thickness from the outer edge to reach an apex and then decreases rapidly to the pupil margin. The thickest point of the iris is at a distance of approximately two-thirds of the radius from the outer edge. This sort of concentric ring around the pupil is the lens. The outer part of the lens is the ciliary area, and the inner part is the pupillary area.

THE REPRESENTATION OF THE LYMPHATIC SYSTEM IN THE IRIS

The condition of the lymphatic system manifests itself in three main circular zones, concentric to the pupil of the eye.

1. An increase in the thickness of the lens corresponds to a stasis of lymph in the abdominal fluids, especially digestive and intestinal fluids.

2. A clear or pigmented area (colors and shades are related to the type and amount of waste stored in the lymphatic system) around the lens corresponds to lymphatic stasis in at least one of the large lymphatic ducts.

3. Debris of various shapes and colors, placed in the fifth outer circular sector of the iris (the sectors are obtained by dividing the iris into six circular sectors from the outer pupillary border), meaning the so-called mesenchymal zone, correspond to problems in the *grundsystem* (see pages 17–24). Sometimes toxins and debris are so abundant that they can create a lymphatic stasis that in effect tries to join the mesenchymal zone with the area around the lens and with the lens itself.

IRIDOPHOTOCHROMOTHERAPY

Iridophotochromotherapy is the stimulation of the iris with beams of light of a specific color and frequency in those areas of the iris that correspond to diseased organs.

It is a therapy developed by Russian researchers at leading Moscow hospitals and disseminated in the West.

We know that the iris is connected to every organ in the body, from where it receives all kinds of information. If the areas corresponding to the discomfort are suitably stimulated, the "way back" can be found and the organ can be repaired.

After many experiments, it was concluded that red light has a stimulating therapeutic effect, blue light a calming effect, and green light a stabilizing effect. It goes without saying that only the part of the iris corresponding to the part of the body to be treated should be treated. Nowadays, each treatment session lasts two or three minutes and is repeated two or three times a week until the desired result is achieved.

Applying this technique to cure circulatory complaints, lymphatic or otherwise, it can be seen that, after about ten sessions, the area corresponding to the lymphatic stasis begins to return to its usual color, and the symptoms related to the complaint begin to disappear.

INDEX

abdomen
lymphatic circulation of, 34–37
lymphatic drainage of, 121–124
Achilles tendon treatment, 147
acne, 73–74
acupoints, and lymphatic system, 190–199
acupuncture needles, 169
Aesculus hippocastanum D1, 167, 199, 212, 213
airways and esophagus, lymphatic circulation of, 42
alfalfa, 215
anabolites, 26
angiology, 76
ankle, treatment of, 148
Ant. tart. 4CH, 191
antagonism, 220
anterior auricular, 56
anterolateral side, treatment of face, 88–97
anti-cellulite therapy, based on vegetable juices, 217
anxiety, 220
Argentum nitricum 5CH, 193
arm
lymphatic circulation of, 43
treatment of, 107–116
arnica, 167
Arnica 5CH, 193
arsenic, 201
arteriosclerosis, 20
arthrosis, 75–76

Aselli, Gaspare, 5
Asian pennywort, 215
aspen, 225
assimilation, 23
atmosphere (Atm), 11–12
auricular lymph nodes
emptying of, 82
second treatment of, 86

Bach, Edward, 219
Bach flowers therapy
emotions and lymphatic stasis, 220–222
lymph and, 219
and lymphatic stasis, 222–226
psyche on disease and vice versa, 220
back massage
as couple, 180
manipulation, 181–182
position, 180–181
back pain treatment
areas to be massaged, 179–180
back massage as couple, 180–182
Bartholin, Thomas, 5
berberis, 167
Betula pubescens D1, 213
bile function, 158
bioelectronic methods, 204
bioflavonoids, 175, 199
black and red currants, 215
blackheads, 74
body versus mind, 159

boldo, 215
brachial station, 54
breast
 lymphatic drainage of, 117–118
 lymphatic stasis of, 177–178
bronchomediastinal duct, 31
bronchomediastinal trunk, 27
buttock region, treatment of,
 129–131

calcium fluoratum, 207
calcium phosphoricum, 209
calcium sulfuricum, 208
calming effect, 230
calorie-only diets, 165
capsule, 50, 51–52
cardiac buoyancy, 10
Carduus marianus, 167
Castanea vesca D1, 197, 212, 213
catabolites, 26
cell, 17–18
 irregular uptake of nutrients by,
  20
cellulite
 external-use creams against,
  214–216
 gemmotherapy recipe against,
  213
 lymphatic self-drainage, 170–173
 menstrual cycle irregularities,
  caused by, 163–164
 overview, 161–163
 prevention and reduction,
  166–169
 reduction of, 68–70
 sedentary lifestyle, due to,
  164–166
cellulitis, 33
centaury, 224
Centella Asiatica, 175, 199
central axillary station, 54

central lymph, 15
cervical region, treatment of,
 104–106
cervical lymph nodes, 84
Chelidonium 5CH, 197
cherry plum, 225
chest wall, lymphatic circulation
 in, 39–40
Chinese acupuncture, 185
ciliary area, 229
circulating lymph, 14–15
clavicle
 drainage areas and related
  disorders, 55
 lymphatic station (position),
  54
Cocculus 5CH, 191
collarbone
 drainage areas and related
  disorders, 55
 lymphatic station (position), 54
comedones, 74
constipation, 158
contraceptive pills, 163
cosmetic surgery, 74, 169
cumin, 215

damiana, 215
daytime sleepiness, 157
debris, 229
deep latero-anterior neck, 58
degeneration, 23
dendritic cells, 52–53
dentistry, 75
diet
 correcting your, 165–166
 ideal daily, 156
digestion, poor, 157
digestive organs, malfunction of,
 163–164
dissociated diet, 165

diuretic, based on vegetable juices, 217
dorsal, treatment of, 127–128
dorsum and instep of foot, treatment of, 149
drainage technique
    movements, 76–77
    number of movements, 77
    perceptions, development of, 78
    phases of each treatment, 79
    pressure techniques, variety of, 78
    rhythm of movements, 78
drowsiness, 157

echinacea, 215
ectasia, formation of, 175
edema, reduction of, 68–70
electrical acupuncture, 168–169
electrical conductivity, 186
electrical fat dissolution. *See* electrolipolysis
electro-acupuncture (EAV), 5, 186–187
electrolipolysis, 168
electrostimulation
    devices, 170
    instruments for, 80
electrotherapy, 168
emboli, 176
emotions
    of anger, 220
    and lymphatic stasis, 220–222
endoplasmic reticulum, 17
endothelium, 26–27
equisetum, 215
escholtzia, 215
esthetic medicine, 72–73
eucalyptus, 75, 191, 215
excretion, 22
eyebrows, treatment of, 92

face
    first treatment of, 88–97
    second treatment of, 98–100
fasting, 165–166
fear (phobias), 220
fenugreek, 215
ferrum phosphoricum, 209
fertilization, 161–162
Ficus carica D1, 197
foot
    dorsum and instep of, treatment of, 149
    interosseous spaces of, treatment of, 150
foot massage, 170–171

gastroesophageal reflux, 193
gemmotherapy, 211–212
    recipe against cellulite, 213
gentian root, 224
glucomannan, 215
grains, 156
grapefruit, 216
grundsystem
    cell, 17–18
    definition, 18
    diagnosis, 21–22
    to lymphatic system, 18–19
    pathologies, 20–21
    phases of, 22–23
    plasma flow in, 19–20
    therapy and healing, 23–24

Hahnemann, Samuel, 201
hallux, treatment of, 151
Hamamelis, 199
head
    lymphatic circulation of, 44–47
    lymphonodal chains of, 82–87
health, restoration of, 23–24
heart, lymphatic circulation of, 42

heather, 226
hemotoxin, 205
hepatobiliary disorder, 220
hiatal hernia, 193
hilum, 50
histolymph. *See also* interstitial
  lymph
  toxins accumulate in, 23
Homeopathy, lymphatic circulation
  and
  history and principles of,
    201–206
  Schüssler salts, 206–209
homeostasis, 10
homotoxicology, 22, 204–205
hydraulic resistance, 26
hypersensitivity, 224

iliac sacs, 6
immune stimulation, 70
immunocompetent cells, 19
impregnation, 23
infarction, 21
inflammation, 22–23
inflammatory bowel problems, 163
inguinal lymph nodes, 56
intercellular fluid, 8
intermediate lymph, 15
internal mammary station, 54
interosseous spaces of foot,
  treatment of, 150
interpectoral lymph nodes, 54
interstitial lymph, 8–14
  appearance and functions, 8
  composition, 8
  histolymph formation from
    capillary circulation, 10–11
  pressure, 11–14
  volume, 9–10
intestinal tract, 27, 31
iodine in seaweed, 217

iridology, brief presentation of,
  227–228
iridophotochromotherapy, 229–230
iris, lymphatic circulation
  represented in
  iridology, brief presentation of,
    227–228
  iridophotochromotherapy,
    229–230
  lymphatic system in, 229
  sructure, 228–229
ischium, 33
ispaghol, 216

Jen Mo, 187
jugular duct, 27, 31
jugular sacs, 6

Kal. carb. 4CH, 193
kalium chloratum, 207
kalium phosporicum, 207
kalium sulfuricum, 208
keloids, 74
knee
  drainage areas and related
    disorders, 63
  lymphatic station (position), 62
  swelling in adolescents, 142–143
  treatment of, 138–141
Krebs cycle, 205

larch, 223
large intestine, lymphatic
  circulation of, 35
leg
  treatment, 144–146
  lymphatic circulation of,
    31–32
  lymphovenous insufficiency in,
    175–177
limbs, stroking, 171–172

liposuction, 169
liver, lymphatic circulation of, 36
lobules, 50
Luffa 5CH, 191
lumbar spine, treatment of,
    127–128
lymph, 1
    and Bach flowers. *See* Bach
        flowers therapy
    classification of, 7
        circulating lymph, 14–15
        interstitial lymph or
            histolymph, 8–14
    make its way through lymphatic
        vessels, 29–30
    and phytotherapy. *See*
        phytotherapy
lymph circulation, 29–30
    abdomen, 34–37
    arms, 43
    head, 44–47
    legs, 31–32
    lymph circulation, 29–30
    lymphatic capillaries, 26–27
    lymphatic capillaries to
        lymphatic ducts, 27–28
    lymphatic pathway, 30
    lymphatic vessels, 28–29
    microcirculation, 25–26
    pelvis, 33–34
    shoulders, 47
    thorax, 37–42
lymph nodes, 1
    appearance under microscope,
        51–53
    dimensions and number, 51
    external appearance, 51
    form, 50
    functions, 49–50
    lymphatic station (position),
        54–63

lymphatic capillaries, 14–15, 19,
    26–27
    to lymphatic ducts, 27–28
    irregular uptake of nutrients by,
        21
lymphatic circulation
    and acupuncture
        Chinese acupuncture, 185
        meridians and lymphatic
            meridian, 187–199
        Voll's electro-acupuncture
            (EAV), 186–187
    represented in iris. *See* iris,
        lymphatic circulation
        represented in
    and well-being
        dream, 157–158
        food, 156–157
        physical and manual activity,
            159–160
        physiological needs, 158
        seven main rules, 155–156
lymphatic drainage
    cellulite prevention and
        reduction, 166
    contraindications, 68
    effects of drainage, 68–72
    general, 67–68
    main clinical indications for,
        72–76
    mechanical and electrical means
        for, 79–80
    technique, 76–79
lymphatic ducts, lymphatic
    capillaries to, 27–28
lymphatic meridian, 187–199
lymphatic pathway, 30
lymphatic points, 22
lymphatic sacs, 6
lymphatic self-drainage, 170

foot, legs, and back,
 manipulations for, 170–173
lymphatic stagnation, 1–2
lymphatic stasis
 and Bach flowers therapy,
 222–226
 of breast, 177–178
 and emotions, 220–222
lymphatic station (position), 54–63
lymphatic system
 formation of, 6–/
 from *grundsystem* to, 18–19
 in iris, representation of, 229
lymphatic vessels, 28–29
lymphocytes, 52
in blood, 7
lymphography, 5
lymphoid tissue centers, in blood, 7
lymphovenous insufficiency, in
 legs, 175–177

macrophages, 49–50
Magn. ph. D6, 195
magnesium-based homeopathic
 product, 178
magnesium phosphoricum, 208
malleoli, treatment of, 148
manual lymphatic drainage, 79
 abdomen, lymphatic drainage of,
 121–124
 Achilles tendon treatment, 147
 ankle and malleoli, treatment
 of, 148
 arm, treatment of, 107–116
 breast, lymphatic drainage of,
 117–118
 cervical and occipital region,
 treatment of, 104–106
 dorsal and lumbar spine,
 treatment of, 127–128

dorsum and instep of foot,
 treatment of, 149
first treatment of face, 88–97
hallux, treatment of, 151
interosseous spaces of foot,
 treatment of, 150
knee
 swelling in adolescents,
 142–143
 treatment of, 138–141
leg treatment, 144–146
occipital region, treatment of,
 101–103
preliminary phase, 82–87
sacral and buttock region,
 treatment of, 129–131
scapula, treatment of, 125–126
second treatment of face, 98–100
tarsus, treatment of, 153
thighs, treatment of, 132–137
thorax, lymphatic drainage of,
 119–120
toes, except the hallux,
 treatment of, 152
massage, 72
 detect areas to be, 179–180
mastoid, 44
mechanical instruments, 79–80
mediastinum, 38
meditation, 159–160
medullary region, 53
melissa, 216
menstrual cycle irregularities,
 caused by, 163–164
Merc. bijod. 5CH, 191
Merc. sol. 5CH, 191
mercury, 201
meridians, 187–199
mesenchymal zone, 229
mesenchyme, 6
mesoderm, 6

mesotherapy, 167
microcirculation, 25–26
  stimulation of, 70–71
milk thistle, 215
mimulus, 225
mineral water (rock water), 219
mitochondria, 17
movements, drainage technique,
  76–77
moxibustion, 187
muriaticum, 207, 209
muscle activation, electrical
  stimulation, 80
muscular drive, lack of, 164

natrium chloratum, 209
natrium phosphoricum, 208
natrum sulfuricum, 207
neck, lymphonodal chains of, 82–87
negative emotions, 219, 222
nettle, 216
neuro-lymphatic treatment
  areas to be massaged, 179–180
  back massage as couple, 180–182
number of movements, drainage
  technique, 77
nutrition, lack of proper, 222

occipital lymph nodes, 83
  drainage areas and related
    disorders, 59
  lymphatic station (position), 58
occipital region, treatment of,
  101–103
Olea europaea D1, 199
oncology, 72
oncotic, 12
orthopedics, 75–76
orthosiphon, 216
osmotic pressure, 10–11
otorhinolaryngology, 75

pancreas, 164
  lymphatic circulation of, 35
papaya, 216
parasternal mammary station, 54
paravertebral lymph nodes, 180
parietal lymph, 28
parotid lymph nodes, 56, 89
  treatment of, 95
Pascal, Blaise, 11
Pecquet's cistern, 28, 62
  lymphatic points of, 189
pectoral muscles, 177–178
pelvis, lymphatic circulation of,
  33–34
perceptions, development of, 78
periosteum, 14–15
peripheral lymph, 14–15
peripheral pump, 14
perpendicular pressure, 181
pharmaceuticals, effect of, 186–187
Phytolacca 5CH, 193
phytotherapy
  cellulite, gemmotherapy recipe
    against, 213
  external-use creams against
    cellulite, 214–216
  gemmotherapy, 211–212
  lymph and, 213
  seaweed, 217
  vegetable juices and WFPS, 217
pilosella, 216
Pistor, Michel, 167
Pituitary and hypothalamus 7CH, 195
plant juices, 217
plasma cells, 52
plasma flow, in *grundsystem*, 19–20
Podophyllum 5CH, 193
popliteal
  drainage areas and related
    disorders, 63
  lymphatic station (position), 62

pressure techniques, variety of, 78
primary lymph nodes, 50
profundus, 56, 86
prostatic point, 203
protein foods, 156
    lack of, 13
psychosomatic problems, 223
Pulsatilla 5CH, 191
putrefaction processes, in intestine, 73

quercus pedunculata D1, 213
quinine, 201

radiant effect, 202
radiation, from medicines, discovery of, 203–204
rapid healing, 70
Reckeweg, H. H., 22, 204
red chestnut, 225
reflexology, 170
rejuvenation, of lymph drainage, 71
relaxation, 72
retina, 228
retroperitoneal sac, 6
Reynaud's syndrome, 20
rhubarb, 216
Rhus tox 5CH, 195
rhythm dysfunctions, 21
rhythm of movements, drainage technique, 78
Ribes nigrum D1, 212
rock rose, 225–226
Rosa canina D1, 212
Rotter's lymph nodes, 54
rubbing, 78

sacral, treatment of, 129–131
sacrolumbar lymphatic circulation, 34

scapula, treatment of, 125–126
Schüssler salts, 206–209
Schüssler, Wilhelm, 206
sclerosing injections, 176
seaweed, 215, 217
sebaceous lymph nodes, 74
secondary lymph nodes, 50
sedentary lifestyle, cellulite due to, 164–166
sexuality, 159–160
shoulders, lymphatic circulation of, 47
silica, 209
small intestine, lymphatic circulation of, 36
social life, 159–160
soledad, 226
Sorbus domestica D1, 197, 212, 213
sports medicine, 76
stabilizing effect, 230
stimulating therapeutic effect, 230
subclavian, 54
subclavian duct, 27, 31
submaxillary lymph nodes, 56
    anterolateral side, treatment of face, 88, 91
    preliminary phase, 85
superficial anterior neck
    drainage areas and related disorders, 61
    lymphatic station (position), 60
superficial latero-anterior neck, 58
superficial lymphatic circulation, 38–39
superior auricular lymph nodes, treatment of, 95
supraclavicular, 54
swelling, reduction of, 68–70
Symphitum 4CH, 193
syphilis, treatment of, 201

taraxacum, 216
targeted treatment. *See* mesotherapy
tarsus, treatment of, 153
temporal auricular lymph nodes, treatment of, 95
temporal lymph nodes, 85
terminal trunks. *See* lymphatic ducts
terminus, 30, 67
termus, 83
thighs, treatment of, 132–137
thinking, 216
thoracic duct, 27, 31, 41
thorax
    lymphatic circulation of, 37–42
    lymphatic drainage of, 119–120
toes, except the hallux, treatment of, 152
tonicity, 71
Torr, 12
Torricelli, Evangelista, 12
Tou Mo, 187
trapezium, lymph nodes of, 84

unexpected grief, 220
upper trapezius region, 47
urogenital region, circulation of, 37

valvular function, 49
varicose veins, 176
vascular hydrodynamic pressure, 10

venoprotectant-based creams, 175
venous capillary, 19
venous hydrostatic pressure, 13–14
venous insufficiency, treatment of, 175
vine, 224
Virchow, Rudolf, 205
visceral lymph, 28
vitamin integrators, 214–216
Vitis vinifera D1, 212
Vodder, Emil, 67
Voll, Reinhold, 22, 186

WALA Magnesit/Mamma comp, 178
WFPS (whole solutions of fresh plants, micronized, frozen, and preserved in alcohol), 217
white chestnut, 223
whiteheads, 74
wild rose, 223
willpower (abulia or stubbornness), 220
witch hazel, 167
worries, 220
worsening, 24

yang, 185
yin, 185
    of liver, 73

Zea mays D1, 212

ABOUT THE AUTHOR

Flavio Gazzola, MD, a specialist in neurology, is an esteemed expert and innovator in natural and holistic medicine. He is renowned for his contributions to acupuncture and traditional Chinese medicine, notably pioneering craniopuncture research in hemiplegia recovery. His work in electro-acupuncture and various bioelectronic diagnostic techniques, such as Ryodoraku, MORA therapy, Vega testing, and computerized somatodensitometry, is prominent in the field. Gazzola's expertise extends to iridology, homeopathy, homotoxicology, phytotherapy, and chirotherapy. As a respected university professor, he has authored numerous books on natural medicine, including *Healing the Incurable* (2006). His website, www.naturalis medicina.it, serves as a comprehensive resource on natural medicine. Gazzola practices in San Donato Milanese in Milan, Italy.